# HELPING YOURSELF WITH WITH NATURAL HEALING

## Lewis Harrison

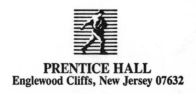

**PRENTICE HALL**
Englewood Cliffs, New Jersey 07632

Prentice-Hall International (UK) Limited, *London*
Prentice-Hall of Australia Pty. Limited, *Sydney*
Prentice-Hall Canada, Inc., *Toronto*
Prentice-Hall Hispanoamericana, S.A., *Mexico*
Prentice-Hall of India Private Limited, *New Delhi*
Prentice-Hall of Japan, Inc., *Tokyo*
Simon & Schuster Asia Pte. Ltd., *Singapore*
Editora Prentice-Hall do Brasil, Ltda., *Rio de Janeiro*

Printed in the United States of America

10   9   8   7   6   5   4   3   2   1

**Library of Congress Cataloging-in-Publication Data**

Harrison, Lewis.
   Helping yourself with natural healing / by Lewis Harrison.
      p.      cm.
   Includes index.
   ISBN 0-13-386749-8          ISBN 0-13-386731-5 (pbk.)
   1. Naturopathy—Popular works.          I.   Title.
RZ440.H365   1988
615.5'--dc19

This book is a reference work based on research by the author. The opinions expressed herein are not necessarily those of or endorsed by the publisher. The directions stated in this book are in no way to be considered as a substitute for consultation with a duly licensed doctor.

ISBN 0-13-386731-5   {PBK}

ISBN 0-13-386749-8

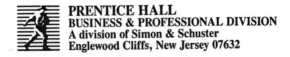
**PRENTICE HALL**
**BUSINESS & PROFESSIONAL DIVISION**
A division of Simon & Schuster
Englewood Cliffs, New Jersey 07632

# Dedication

*To those who supported my vision to create a work that would make a difference in people's lives. My deepest appreciation to Nelsa Padin, Dr. Daniel J. Wiener, my parents Dorothy and Harold Harrison and to my guide and teacher Maharaj Charan Singh Ji.*

# Acknowledgments

To the visionaries, pioneers, writers, physicians, journalists and other dedicated individuals who have made great contributions to creating and maintaining the evolution and growth of the natural healing, self healing and naturopathic movements throughout the world;

Dr. Issac Jennings, Russel Thacker Trall M.D., Henry Lindhlar M.D., Bernarr MacFadden, Benedict Lust N.D., John Tilden M.D., John Harvey Kellog M.D., Alice Chase M.D., Herbert Shelton, Sylvester Graham, Juan Amon Wilkins, Jesse Mercer Gehman, N.D., Paavo Airola, N.D., J. I. Rodale, John Christopher N.D., Adelle Davis, Dr. Carlton Fredericks, Ann Wigmore, Viktoras Kulvinskas, Gary Null. Special thanks to Vincent Collura, my first teacher for introducing me this work.

My special thanks, to the researchers shamans, healers researchers and staff and unamed individuals who responded to my requests for information especially Leslie Kasloff for his assistance in organizing the chapter on the Bach Flower Remedies, and Sara Vogeler for her assistance on the chapter on Body Therapies;

Special thanks to the following people and companies who provided me with information: Tom Johnson, The Heritage Store, Ilene Bryan, at Mega Food (TM), National Enzyme Company, Mr. George Higashida of Sun Chlorella California Inc., Terrace International Distributors, Inc., Irving Chase of the Henry Thayer Company, Da Vinci Laboratories, Jeff Traister of Tyson & Associates, Natural Organics Inc., Volunteer Lawyers For The Arts, and Barbara Steiner, Staff assistant at the News Office for the Medical Area at Harvard University.

# Contents

27 • Be Sure to Exercise! / 27 • Range-of-Motion Exercises / 27 • Tai Chi and Hatha Yoga / 28 • A Word of Warning About Exercising / 28 • Hydrotherapy and Other Techniques / 28 • Homeopathy / 29 • Edgar Cayce Remedies / 29 • The Value of Rest and Relaxation / 29 • Control Pain Through Visualization Techniques / 30 • Also of Interest / 30 • How Dorothy H. Found Relief From Osteoarthritis / 31 • For Your Information / 32

# An Introduction to Natural Healing

Natural healing and orthodox medicine are often viewed as opposing forces; as two different systems at war with each other. Yet, natural healing and orthodox medicine actually share the same basic goal: to make people feel better. However, there are many major, fundamental differences in how these two approaches attempt to reach that common goal.

In natural healing, for example, nutrition plays a central role, along with the emotions, spirituality, and the environment. Often ignored as "folk medicine," holistic approaches offer many ways to achieve health.

On the other hand, orthodox medicine has lost touch with the role and the value of nutrition in health care. It advocates, instead, a strong intervention approach to health care. In orthodox medicine, treatment is limited mainly to medication and surgery! The result is that the drugs and medical procedures used to cure an illness can often, ironically, cause disability, sometimes death.

Although the natural health professional is willing to use virtually any means of diagnosing and treating illness—yes, even medication and surgery—the natural healer does not *rely exclusively* on such extreme, risky approaches. The reason is simple: instead of analyzing and then treating one part of the body, the natural healer analyzes the entire body, including the mind and the spirit (thus the word *holistic*). That is THE difference between natural healing and orthodox medicine.

*Helping Yourself with Natural Healing* offers you alternatives to traditional medical treatments for many common problems—presenting techniques that may be new to you for healing yourself. The remedies are safe and natural. *Helping Yourself with Natural Healing* is designed to help you tap into your body's profound potential for self-healing and balance. After all, good health is the *normal* human condition.

See a physician in any case of illness. The remedies in this volume should be shown to a physician before attempting self-treatment.

# 1

# Aging

Everyone knows that aging is inevitable. But contrary to popular opinion, the mental and physical decline associated with aging is *not* inevitable, according to recent research studies.

Perhaps as much as half of the functional physical decline that takes place between age 30 and age 70 is the result of *disuse* of the body, not of aging itself. Similarly, according to other studies, essential areas of human intelligence do not diminish among older people who are healthy. In fact, certain types of intelligence actually increase!

As we age, our body systems do slow down, and perhaps this is most noticeable in our digestive system. Elderly people often experience a decrease in the sense of taste and smell. They have more difficulty absorbing essential nutrients—a process made worse because at the same time, they tend to take in fewer nutrients. Many elderly people take medications that hamper food absorption, diminish nutrient metabolism, and upset their bodies' nutritional balance. For people over 65, calcium absorption decreases, and diarrhea or constipation may occur more often.

Let's take a closer look at what you can do to offset the negative effects of aging on the digestive system.

## Eat Less, Live Longer

Want to add years to your life? Follow a diet that includes all the essential nutrients (of course), but about 30 percent fewer calories than are needed to maintain your normal body weight. Such a diet can lessen the possibility of heart and kidney diseases, cancer, and arthritis.

An eminent immunologist, Dr. Robert A. Good of the Oklahoma Medical Research Foundation, goes one step further. He says that *"even genetically determined diseases* may be modified or even entirely prevented by limiting the protein, calories or fat content of the diet.''* [Jane E. Brody, "Eating Less May Be the Key to Living Beyond 100 Years,"* *New York Times,* June 8, 1982.]

Here are some tips to help ensure that you *do* get all the essential nutrients in your diet.

## Get the Most Out of Nutrients

Because nutrients can be so helpful in slowing down the aging process, you should consider all these tips.

• Whenever you cook vegetables in soups, add a little apple cider vinegar. Reason: the apple cider vinegar draws out the beneficial calcium.

• Eat plenty of dried peas and beans, pumpkin seeds, brussel sprouts, oatmeal, peanuts, brazil nuts, pecans, sunflower seeds, filberts, walnuts, almonds, and sesame seeds to increase your intake of zinc.

Zinc is a trace mineral that is essential for many fundamental processes, including the proper digestion of carbohydrates, protein metabolism, the production of RNA and DNA, the transport of carbon dioxide in the blood, elimination of carbon dioxide from the lungs, insulin production, and more.

• Avoid coffee. It can block your body's ability to absorb zinc.

• Minimize the use of oils in cooking and preparing foods. Excessive use of polyunsaturated oils can contribute to premature aging.

• Whenever you cook acidic foods (for example, tomatoes, citrus fruits, vinegar, and cranberries), use a cast-iron pot. This is a simple way to increase the content of iron in the food you're cooking.

• Do your dentures bother you when you eat certain foods? If so, then try grating your vegetables to soften them. Also, increase your intake of steamed fruits and vegetables. Cottage cheese, yogurt, and other low-fat milk products are easy to eat. They are also a low-cost source of protein and calcium.

• Include plenty of garlic, onion, and cabbage in your diet. These foods are excellent sources of L-Cysteine, an amino acid that blocks the actions of harmful chemicals in polluted air and in tobacco smoke, which can cause wrinkling of the skin.

• Add fiber to your diet. There is evidence that diverticulitis, gallbladder disease, and colon cancer may be directly related to the amount of fiber in your diet.

• To avoid poor muscular function, which is very common in the elderly, eat potassium-rich foods. Add beans to your diet, and fresh fruits, such as bananas, apricots, oranges, cantaloupe, raisins, figs, and dates; and vegetables, especially broccoli, potatoes, and peas. For snacking, try almonds, pecans, olives, and molasses.

• Do not overlook your need for protein. Older people require about the same amount of protein as young adults.

• For vitamin A, be sure to eat green leafy vegetables and fresh fruit. Vitamin A is essential for healthy eyes, ears, lungs, nose, throat, skin, glands, mucous membranes, and so on. Vitamin A also protects against the effects of various air pollutants. Sources of vitamin A include:

**Vegetables:**

| | | |
|---|---|---|
| Beet tops | Broccoli | Chicory |
| Collard greens | Endive | Escarole |
| Dandelion greens | Kale | Carrots |
| String beans | Swiss chard | Tomatoes |
| Mustard greens | Green peas | Red peppers |
| Sweet potatoes | Watercress | Yellow squash |

Lettuce (Boston, bib, and romaine only)

**Fruits:**

| | | |
|---|---|---|
| Apricots | Avocados | Bananas |
| Cherries | Oranges | Prunes |
| Cantaloupes | Papayas | Yellow peaches |

• Avoid using alcohol. The old saying that claims drinking "in moderation" is beneficial has no merit. Alcohol adversely affects too many of your body's important routine functions. (See the section entitled "Alcohol Use and Abuse.")

• Perhaps you've already heard all the claims about the power of lecithin in the treatment of certain disorders associated with aging. Well, they're usually true! Lecithin has been proven effective in lowering cholesterol levels in the bloodstream and in the treatment of atherosclerosis and heart disease. Numerous studies also show that it may be valuable in the treatment of neurological disorders such as Parkinson's disease and tardive dyskinesia (incomplete movement of voluntary muscles, usually in the face).

## Three Key Tips

1. Use fresh whole foods and prepare them simply, without boiling, frying, or overcooking.

2. Choose foods that are high in fiber, low in fat, high in unrefined complex carbohydrates, and moderate in protein.

3. Use cultured-milk products such as kefir, buttermilk, or yogurt. These will help maintain the normal bacterial flora in the intestines and aid in digestion.

## Use Supplements to Live Longer

Except for calcium, most physicians see no need for nutritional supplements in the diets of the elderly. There is, however, a wealth of evidence that proves otherwise. Many supplements will be especially beneficial to you as you get older.

*Vitamin E.* Take vitamin E, for example. As you get older, your immune system may become less effective. Studies show that vitamin E helps to delay the slowdown in the immune system. In fact, Russian researchers claim that large doses of vitamins A and E can increase strength, smooth facial wrinkles, eliminate headaches, restore gray hair to its natural color, and generally slow down the aging process.

Vitamin E reduces the oxygen requirement of tissues and thereby "saves" oxygen. The saved oxygen is then passed on to the brain cells.

*Iron and $B_{12}$.* As you age, your gastric system tends to secrete less hydrochloric acid. This is one of the reasons you should supplement your diet with iron and $B_{12}$.

*CoQ.* The supplement coenzyme Q10 (also known as "CoQ" or "ubiquinone") has a number of anti-aging effects. One effect is that it helps increase the tolerance for exercise in people who do a lot of sitting. Coenzyme Q10 also helps protect the immune system from age-related problems, is a helpful treatment for periodontal disease, and is prevention against the toxic (poisonous) effects of many drugs used to treat cancer, hypertension, and other diseases common among the elderly.

*Lecithin.* In early studies, lecithin appeared helpful to three of seven people suffering from Alzheimer's disease. Specifically, lecithin improved their speech, their ability to understand information quickly and clearly, and their ability to learn. When lecithin supplements stopped, so did the improvements.

*$B_{12}$.* Senility has been associated with deficiencies in all the B complex vitamins—especially folic acid, thiamine ($B_1$), $B_{12}$, and niacin ($B_3$)—as well as vitamins C and E and choline.

*Niacin.* An aid to certain circulatory problems, niacin can thin the blood and prevent clumping or sludging of blood cells.

*Zinc.* A zinc deficiency can result in a loss of taste and smell; a loss which, in turn, often can produce a domino effect: because of this loss of taste and smell, people have less of a desire to eat; their poor eating habits then lead to poor nutrition; and poor nutrition, of course, eventually leads to a number of other ailments. You can see once again, therefore, the importance of zinc in your diet!

*L-Cysteine.* L-Cysteine, which was mentioned earlier, is an amino acid that blocks the actions of harmful air pollutants, including tobacco smoke, which can promote wrinkling of the skin.

## Adding Herbs for Alertness and Concentration

The herb ginseng appears to have tremendous natural healing powers. In certain studies, for example, elderly patients who used high-grade ginseng for a period of three months showed:

- Less rigidity than before.
- Increased alertness.
- Increased ability to concentrate.
- Improved visual-motor coordination.
- Improved ability to understand abstract concepts.
- Improved respiration.
- Greater ease in performing physical tasks.

Other herbs are also helpful. The juice of young green barley plants (sold in dehydrated form in the United States as *green magma*) can normalize and rejuvenate cells and tissues, repair damaged DNA, restore cellular activity, and prevent tissue from aging.

Another herb, Fo Ti, is of Chinese origin. Fo Ti helps memory and reduces depression.

*The Amazing Ginkgo Leaf.* Ginkgo biloba extract has been found to be of great value for those suffering from various geriatric complaints due to lack of circulation to the brain. These symptoms include vertigo, tinnitus (ringing in the ears), short term memory loss, lack of vigilance, and depression.

## Aroma Therapy for Continued Health

As you seek other ways to slow the aging process and live longer and better, consider *aroma therapy*, another helpful treatment. Aroma therapy is the use of essences to treat physical or psychological disorders.

For example, oil of rosemary is traditionally used to help improve memory. For relieving insomnia and extreme nervousness, "sedating oils" such as cajuput, chamomile, melissa, and peppermint are useful. The specific application depends on the individual aromatic essence. It may be inhaled or taken orally; or it can be applied as a compress, massaged onto body parts directly, or added to your bath oil.

## Exercise for the Elderly

Exercise is, of course, an important aspect of holistic healing. In fact, exercise is not a luxury, as many people think; it is a necessity! Exercising is essential for good health and a high quality of living. It is a means of releasing emotional tensions and achieving physical balance. A "health program" that does not specifically address the issue of exercise is useless because it overlooks a major therapeutic factor.

Exercise has many benefits. Among others, exercise helps to:

- Lower blood pressure.
- Control weight.
- Increase or reduce blood sugars (of special value to diabetics).
- Improve your physical appearance and sense of well-being by reducing flab, improving your skin tone, and giving you a more restful night's sleep.
- Reduce risk of cardiovascular disease.
- Increase your capacity to work.
- Improve your blood and respiratory functions.
- Give you denser (stronger) bones.
- Enhance clear thinking and reduce your susceptibility to depression.
- Give you more energy and stamina.
- Improve your self-image.
- Increase your resistance to high blood pressure, diabetes, arthritis, osteoporosis, and some forms of cancers.

Are these benefits worth working for? You bet they are! The exercises that are especially appropriate for older people are yoga, tai chi, swimming, dancing, bike riding, and brisk walking (3 to 5 miles a day or as recommended by your physician). These exercises offer the greatest benefits with the least amount of physical discomfort, stress, or injury.

Needless to say, however, there are a number of *dos* and *don'ts* associated with exercising.

### Don't Exercise . . .

- Without your physician's approval.
- When you are taking medications.
- After drinking alcohol (the result can be dehydration or an irregular heartbeat).

- If you have an injury of some kind.
- If you have a history of high blood pressure or some chronic illness.

### Do Exercise . . .

- *Regularly*! The greatest culprits of exercise are the words "I don't have time" and "I'm too tired now."
- Before your meals. Early morning or midevening are the best times. If you must exercise during the day, exercise at least 90 minutes after your last meal.
- After meditating or breathing quietly to relax your body and calm your mind.
- After warming up for a few minutes.
- In an encouraging environment. Do everything possible to avoid boredom. Play music, vary your routine, find a friend who will join you, avoid distractions, and so on.

*A Word About Yoga.* Hatha-yoga is a system of stretching and breathing exercises, meditation and visualization techniques, and other techniques used to bring about physical, mental, and emotional balance. Often simply called *yoga*, it is a powerful self-healing tool, not a spiritual or religious philosophy, as many people incorrectly think.

The yoga stretching movements are performed in a slow, methodical way, reducing the chance of injury. Some of the stretching movements are simple to perform, even for beginners. If you practice the movements properly and regularly, you can make your spine elastic, tone your muscles, firm your skin, and improve poor posture. As with all exercise programs, begin slowly and proceed carefully.

## Tips to Remember

In addition to all we have discussed so far, by observing the following guidelines, you can contribute positively to the aging process.

- Maintain friendships and make new friends. Avoid being alone except for meditation times and planned solitude.
- Avoid excessive exposure to the sun and you will help avoid premature wrinkling and premature aging.
- Do not ignore high blood pressure; monitor it carefully. Elderly people have been known to faint after meals because their blood pressure dropped after they ate. Blood pressure may also drop—*as much as 20 points*—when elderly people stand up suddenly. ["Mealtime May Be a Factor in Fainting in Aged," *New York Times*, July 14, 1983.]
- Listen to pleasant music often, with friends, family or alone. Music therapy has been found very effective for helping memory recall (by encouraging elderly people to recognize different musical instruments), for increasing the effectiveness of dance and movement therapy, and for communicating with people who feel isolated.
- Use stainless steel or other nonaluminum cookware. Researchers have found traces of aluminum in the brains of victims of Alzheimer's disease. Although the cause of Alzheimer's is not known, finding traces of aluminum in the brain is not typical. Is there a danger of using aluminum cookware, as many natural healers have warned for years? Or does the aluminum come from those natural foods, food additives, and ant-

acids that contain aluminum? We do not know, but to be on the safe side, avoid cooking with aluminum cookware.

## For Your Information

The following resources may be helpful to you in changing—or just *improving*—your life style.

Center for the Study of Aging
706 Madison Avenue
Albany, NY 12208
(519) 465-6927

Gray Panthers
311 South Juniper Street
Suite 601
Philadelphia, PA 19107
(215) 545-6555

American Association for Retired People
555 Madison Avenue
New York, NY 10022
(212) 758-1411

Friends & Relatives of the
    Institutionalized Aged, Inc.
440 East 26 Street
New York, NY 10010
(212) 481-4422

Lifeline Systems, Inc.*
839 Beacon Street
Boston, MA 02215
(617) 267-2693

For more information about ginkgo biloba extract, contact

Global Marketing Associates
435 Brannan Street
San Francisco, CA 94107
(415) 495-8524

---

* Lifeline Systems offers a beeper-system telephone attachment that elderly people living alone can use to get help quickly in an emergency.

# 2

# Alcohol Use
# and Abuse

Despite advertisers' claims to the contrary, alcoholic beverages simply do not contain "the finest ingredients," regardless of what goes into the manufacturing process. In fact, the list of *naturally occurring substances* found in wines includes chemicals, gases, minerals, even small amounts of methanol. Add to this list all the ingredients that the winery contributes: hydrogen peroxide, activated charcoal, calcium sulfate, propylene glycol, sulfur dioxide, potassium bicarbonate, oak extract, and on and on.

The result is not exactly thirst-quenching! Furthermore, note these findings concerning the use of alcohol:

• Regular intake of alcohol can lower your sex drive; abuse of alcohol destroys essential male sex hormones.

• If you drink and smoke at the same time, your risk of cancer increases *fifteenfold*!

• Alcohol intake may contribute to a number of nutritional deficiencies.

• Certain birth defects occur as the result of the sperm damage associated with alcohol use.

• Rectal cancer has been linked to beer drinking.

• Low blood sugar (hypoglycemia) may result from alcohol use.

• You have a greater risk of hearing loss as a result of alcohol use. The muscle in the middle ear that contracts to protect the eardrum from loud noises works less effectively when there is alcohol in your system.

## Alcohol Use and Nutrition

Besides being overloaded with a number of frightening substances, the bald fact is that alcoholic beverages are high in calories and low in nutrients. Also, alcohol use is directly responsible for a loss of vitamin C in the body, and this loss of vitamin C may contribute, in turn, to other nutritional deficiencies.

Not surprisingly, then, alcoholics are commonly lacking in vitamin C, zinc, and magnesium. Further, alcoholics may have difficulty absorbing thiamine, folic acid, and vitamin $B_{12}$. As a result, they may be predisposed to:

| | |
|---|---|
| Hypoglycemia | Headaches |
| Chronic fatigue | Ulcers |
| Adrenal insufficiency | Cirrhosis of the liver |

But the list doesn't end there: in addition, alcohol can alter male sexual behavior by destroying essential male sex hormones, and it can increase the possibility of breast, skin, and thyroid cancer.

## Fast to Cleanse Toxins From Your System

The first step on the road to recovery from the effects of alcohol is to cleanse the system of toxins. The goal of fasting is to rid the body of metabolic wastes, toxins, and other poisonous substances accumulated through the use of alcohol. At the same time as it cleanses, a juice fast also provides enzymes which are valuable to the healing and rehabilitation process. Be aware that all fasts beyond 2 to 3 days should be conducted under the supervision of a health professional familiar with the benefits and limitations of fasting programs.

Fast on juices for 10 to 14 days:

• Use only freshly extracted fruit and vegetable juices. Canned and bottled juices are of little or no value in a juice therapy program. Effective juice therapy requires fresh pressed juices because they are high in enzymes and nutrients. Virtually all the authorities on this healing approach agree that the processing that takes place in the processing and packaging of canned and bottled juices (including pasteurization) has been found to reduce both of these essential factors. Check that all green vegetables have a rich, full color. Avoid iceberg lettuce, blanched celery, etc.

• Drink the juice immediately after you extract it. Do not store or refrigerate the juice for later use.

• Juice therapy formula #18 can be included among the juice mixtures that are especially healthy. Or you can squeeze ten lemons in two quarts of water; drink a glass every two hours. Another helpful drink is a mixture of seven ounces of green leafy vegetable juice and seven ounces of beet juice combined with two ounces of dandelior juice. Take this combination twice daily.

Proper fasting will help your body eliminate waste matter through your bowels, skin, lungs, kidneys, and so on. To aid in the process, you should also try steam baths, stretching exercises, and saunas.

The next step after fasting is to establish a diet that will replenish the nutrients your body has lost and help you return to your normal healthy state.

## Diet Your Way Back to Health

Once your body is cleansed of metabolic wastes, toxins, and other poisons, you are ready to begin a *modified raw food diet*. The diet must provide adequate calories and must be high in both protein and the B vitamins. (Protein is especially important if cirrhosis of the liver has occurred.) Later, you will see how to supplement the diet to provide the necessary amino acids, vitamins, and minerals.

A modified raw food diet is described on page 00.

## Use Supplements to Recover from the Effects of Alcohol

For a number of reasons, dietary changes alone are unlikely to offset the effects of long-term alcohol use. The nutritional deficiencies found in alcohol abusers are so pervasive that supplements of amino acids, vitamins, and minerals appear mandatory. Here's why.

Alcohol users typically have an imbalance in their amino acid metabolism, and amino acids are essential for many, many different aspects of your health. Often called "the building blocks of protein," amino acids make up over 75 percent of your total body solids. As a result, alcohol abusers require combination-free amino acids—especially L-Tryptophan—to correct this imbalance.

A "combination-free" amino acid is one that is not combined with other nutrients or other amino acids. This need for combination-free amino acids is most apparent in those individuals who experience depression and aggression after they stop drinking. In fact, those individuals with histories of extremely aggressive behavior may need a health professional to administer L-Tryptophan.

To establish a program of supplements, consider these facts:

• Vitamin A helps reduce the upper-respiratory infections that are common among alcohol abusers.

• A vitamin B complex reduces neuritis, delirium tremens (the "shakes"), and pellagra, all three of which are common among alcohol abusers.

• Choline assists in the decomposition of fats in the liver and helps maintain healthy kidneys, often damaged through alcohol abuse.

• Vitamin C, zinc, iron, magnesium, potassium—all are deficient among alcohol abusers.

• When used together, vitamin C, L-Cysteine, and thiamine provide protection against acetaldehyde, a metabolite of alcohol that is more toxic than alcohol itself. [*Agents and Actions*, Volume 5, No. 2, 1975.]

• In a few studies, L-Glutamine was found effective in reducing the craving for alcohol.

• According to many nutritionists, anti-oxidants may prevent hangovers and relieve the long-term toxic effects of alcohol. The most effective anti-oxidants are vitamin C, vitamin $B_1$, Cysteine, and L-Glutathione.

## Add Herbs to End the Craving

Herbs, too, can be very helpful in the recovery process. Taken every two hours, chaparral capsules will help clean the liver and reduce the craving for alcohol. Other helpful herbs include skullcap, angelica, cayenne, and chamomile.

Mix this tea to help increase elimination:

2 parts Plantain
1 part Parsley
1 part Yellow dock
1 part Fennel

## Hydrotherapy Speeds Recovery

To contribute to a faster recovery, try warm-water enemas or alternating hot and cold showers.

Especially effective for dealing with alcohol abuse is dry brushing before and after showers and baths. Take a natural plant fiber brush, a loofah or a coarse grade natural sponge (these are available in health food stores, drug or hardware stores). Begin with the soles of your feet and brush vigorously in a circular motion. Then massage every part of your body in the following sequence: feet, legs, hands, arms, back, abdomen, cheek, neck and face. This will increase the circulation and remove dead skin, while producing a refreshed and energizing feeling. Be careful not to brush too hard. After the dry brush massage, take alternating hot and cold showers as described in the hydrotherapy section of the appendix.

## For Your Information

Alcoholics Anonymous, a well-known nonprofit organization with chapters throughout the country, can provide much help and support to alcohol abusers and their families.

Alcoholics Anonymous
P.O. Box 459
Grand Central Station
New York, NY 10163
(212) 686-1100

# 3

# Allergies

What are allergies? For our purposes, we can loosely define *allergy* as an abnormal reaction to a food or an environmental substance. Why "abnormal"? Because the same food or substance does *not* bother most people!

An allergic reaction results because the body identifies this food or substance as an intruder, as a potentially dangerous attacker, and then reacts to the intrusion. To respond to the "threat" of, say, milk, the body sets its defense system into action when the milk enters the body. Of course, there is no reason the body *should* react to milk, but it does anyway; thus, "abnormal" applies.

As soon as the milk combines with a certain antibody in our blood, the body mounts a counterattack by producing the chemical *histamine*. It is this chemical, histamine, that causes the typical symptoms of allergic reactions, such as swollen blood vessels, inflamed skin, tightened air passages, and itching of the eyes. All this discomfort for what is essentially a "false alarm"!

## A Widespread Problem

Many foods, including many *common* foods, can cause allergic reactions. Among the top offenders are:

| | | |
|---|---|---|
| Cow's milk | Wheat | Corn |
| Eggs | Nuts | Seafood |
| Chocolate | Alcohol | Citrus fruits |

Recent studies show that allergy-like reactions and problems are not limited to foreign substances—known as *allergens*—combining with antibodies alone. Allergens may also react with other blood elements. Add to this the fact that there are many more conditions caused by allergies and food sensitivity that are not recognized as such, and you begin to see the scope of the problem.

In fact, allergic reactions may be the most frequently unrecognized cause of illness in the United States! A few of the many, many allergy-induced disorders are:

### General Disorders

| | |
|---|---|
| Anemia | Hearing and ear problems |
| Arthritis | Hoarseness |
| Bloating | Hyperactivity |
| Bursitis | Inflammation |
| Canker sores | Joint pain and swelling |
| Chills | Fatigue |
| Circulatory problems | Menstrual difficulties |
| Coughing | Nosebleeds |
| Cramps | Rectal pain and itching |
| Dandruff | Urinary problems |
| Depression | Vaginal itching and burning |
| EKG changes | Vision and eye problems |
| Headaches | Vomiting |
| Heart pain and palpitations | Wheezing |

### Gastrointestinal Disorders

| | |
|---|---|
| Flatulence | Colic |
| Colitis | Nausea |
| Diarrhea | Ulcers |

### Respiratory Disorders

| | |
|---|---|
| Asthma | Bronchitis |
| Pneumonia | |

### Skin Disorders

| | |
|---|---|
| Contact dermatitis | Itching |
| Eczema | Rashes |
| Hives | Welts |

Even this partial listing is obviously impressive in pointing to allergic reactions as a major cause of illnesses and disorders.

## What Increases Your Susceptibility?

Various factors may increase your susceptibility to allergies, including:

- Heredity
- Brain sensitivity to food. Many people eat in response to depression or anxiety. The opposite may also be true: people may become anxious or depressed in response to eating. Such a response is a direct result of brain sensitivity to certain foods.

• Repetitious eating patterns. Many nutritionists and physicians report that people who constantly eat the same foods on a regular basis over an extended period of time can develop a sensitivity or allergy to those foods.

• Care during infancy. Breast-fed children have fewer allergies than bottle-fed children. Also, if infants are fed highly antigenic foods (such as cow's milk and eggs) during the first few months after birth, then food sensitivity is likely to develop, especially if the infants have a hereditary disposition toward allergies.

• Weak adrenal gland function.

• Low digestive enzymes and poor nutrient absorption.

• Environmental conditions (weather, temperature).

• Photosensitivity to drugs and chemicals. Many people react allergically to the combination of sunlight with certain drugs and chemicals (whether the drugs or chemicals are taken orally or administered topically). As a result, the skin parts exposed to the sun may show an intense sunburn, an itchy or painful rash, redness or swelling, or some similar symptom. Most photosensitivity reactions do not last long. They generally end when you stop using the chemical or stop the exposure to ultraviolet light.

## Diagnosing Your Allergies

There are several methods for diagnosing your allergies. The most common and most effective are described here.

*The Four-Day Food-Rotation Plan.* Following this plan, as the name broadly hints, you eat a particular food in modest amounts *every four days*. As you do so, keep a detailed diary of (1) which foods you eat; (2) when you eat each food item; (3) how much you eat of each item; and (4) your reactions, if any, to each food, even seemingly insignificant reactions.

In this way, you can better isolate specific symptoms, associate the reactions with certain foods, and then avoid those foods. Although this method for identifying food sensitivity is obviously inexpensive, it is not as accurate as other procedures. To improve its accuracy, this plan is often used together with Dr. Coca's Pulse Test. [Arthur F. Coca, *The Pulse Test*, New York: Lyle Stuart, 1967.]

*RAST.* The *radioallergosorbent test*, simply known as *RAST*, is an inhalant test that determines antibody levels for specific allergens that might be present in your bloodstream. RAST not only identifies which inhalants cause allergic responses but also shows the degree of severity of each response. Therefore, it is especially helpful in identifying the appropriate treatment. RAST results are more specific than results from cytotoxic testing.

*Cytotoxic (Food) Testing.* In this lab test, a doctor or technician uses a blood sample to test the reaction of your white blood cells to 150 (or more) different foods. Using a microscope, the doctor or technician determines your allergy to foods by observing how severely each food destroys white blood cells.

## Use Supplements to Combat Allergies

Some supplements are very helpful in fighting off allergic responses.

• Vitamins A, B complex, C, and E are especially effective for hay fever sufferers. Vitamin C seems to have a powerful antihistamine quality that reduces the symptoms of hay fever.

• Bioflavonoids and pantothenic acid are also helpful in reducing hay fever symptoms.

• Selenium and glutathione are anti-oxidants (like vitamins C and E) that help provide relief from allergies.

• Acidophilus (*lactobacillus acidophilus*) is a bacterial strain that has numerous healing properties, especially concerning the immune system. High-potency strains of acidophilus (1) build strong immunities, (2) maintain intestinal acid balance, and (3) inhibit the growth of unfriendly bacteria in the urinary tract, as well as in the respiratory and reproductive systems. In addition to its specific usefulness in fighting allergic reactions, acidophilus is a very useful general healing tool. Acidophilus is especially recommended when you are taking antibiotics.

NOTE: If you have a milk allergy, begin taking acidophilus in very small doses and monitor any reactions you may have. Better yet, use an acidophilus product cultured from a nonmilk source.

To reduce the effect of food sensitivity, you may find the following program useful:

• One hour before mealtime, take:
  1 level teaspoon of sodium ascorbate powder (vitamin C)
  3 to 5 100-milligram bromelain tablets
  A digestive enzyme product
  Approximately 15 milligrams of free amino acids
• With your meals, take:
  100 to 250 milligrams of vitamin $B_6$ (pyridoxine)
  Five 100-milligram tablets of $B_2$ (riboflavin) throughout the day
  500 milligrams of pantothenic acid

## What About Reactions to Supplements?

Allergic reactions to supplements are probably reactions to the various additives that supplements may contain, not the active ingredients themselves. While the active ingredients may be very beneficial, the benefits may be offset by additives.

• Dyes
• Coloring agents
• Artificial flavors (especially in vitamin products for children)
• Preservatives (in tablets, usually benzoates)
• Sulfates (for example, ferrous sulfate)
• Binders, fillers, lubricants, and inert substances
• Coal tars
• Sugar, starch, salt
• Animal-derived stearates
• Pesticide residues
• Fillers and coatings

For a source of nonallergenic vitamins and supplements, see "For Your Information" at the end of this section.

## Juice Therapy

Twice a day, drink this 18-ounce mixture: 12 ounces of carrot juice, 3 ounces of beet juice, and 3 ounces of cucumber juice.

## Herbal Remedies

Many herbs effectively combat allergy symptoms. Among the herbs most commonly used are the following:

| | |
|---|---|
| Mullein leaves | Echinacea root |
| Bayberry bark | Rosehips |
| Red Clover blossoms | Comfrey |
| Goldenseal root | Juniper |

## Aroma Therapy

Aroma therapy can be very effective for hay fever. Try essence of hyssop to relieve common hay fever symptoms. Hyssop should be used here by vapor dispersal through the room.

## Homeopathy

Three homeopathic remedies are especially recommended for hay fever:

*Arsenicum.* Take arsenicum for hay fever accompanied by painful, violent sneezing, a profuse watery discharge, a burning sensation on the lips, and a feeling of worry and restlessness.

*Dulcamara.* Try dulcamara for hay fever accompanied by swollen, watery eyes, a runny, stuffed-up nose, and chills (despite the fact that the skin may actually feel hot).

*Nux Vomica.* Use nux vomica when hay fever symptoms include: long, intense sneezing spells, irritated nose—stuffy at night, and eyes and face that feel hot while the rest of the body feels chilled.

## Tissue Salts

*A Word About Tissue Salts.* Tissue salts are inorganic substances that are normally present in the body in very small quantities. The basic theory of tissue salt therapy is that when the normal quantity of a particular tissue salt is low for any reason, the body is imbalanced. To regain a balanced state, you must intake the deficient tissue salt, which will allow the body to readily assimilate the needed tissue salt.

For hay fever, try these three tissue salts in combination: magnesium phosphate, sodium chloride, and silicic oxide. See Appendix for further information on Homeopathy.

## Tips to Remember

For extra protection against the effects of allergies:

• Isolate the cause of your allergy. Don't overlook the obvious. You may be reacting to the spray cleaner you use, your pet's dander, the dust of roaches, and so on.

• "Inspect your basement for moldiness and dampness. Look around the kitchen for cockroaches. Examine every air conditioner and humidifier for molds and, while you're at it, clean all the filters. Check the tops of electric light bulbs, the grills of heating vents, and all venetian blinds for dust. Slap the cushions on the couches and chairs to see if they give off dust and feathers." This is the advice of Dr. Murray Dworetzky, Physician-in-Chief of the Allergy Clinic at New York Hospital-Cornell Medical Center. [Donald Robinson, "When Home Can Hurt You," *Parade Magazine*, November 24, 1985, p. 8.]

• Clean all dust with a damp cloth or mop, not a vacuum cleaner. Vacuum cleaners spread dust with their exhausts.

• Substitute electric heat for gas heat, if possible.

• Brush your teeth with a combination of baking soda and salt. You may be reacting to something in your toothpaste (even a natural toothpaste).

## How Susan R. Attacked Her Allergy Problems

For no apparent reason, every afternoon about 1 o'clock, Susan R. became very tired. An account executive for a large New York City firm, she suffered from red, itchy skin and continuous sinus problems. After a year of trying various over-the-counter skin creams and sinus medications, Susan realized that allergies could be the cause of her symptoms, and she was right!

First, Susan began a cleansing and healing program. For three days, her only nutrition consisted of a mixture of 32 ounces of carrot, beet, and cucumber juice. In addition, she drank as much as she wanted of two blood purifiers: (1) distilled water with lemon juice and (2) red clover tea.

Then, at the end of three days, she began the food rotation plan and discovered that she was sensitive to meat, cow's milk, cheese (but not to yogurt and buttermilk), wheat, tomatoes, and corn. Susan eliminated these foods from her diet, as well as foods that contained artificial colors, flavors, and preservatives. Also, she went for a colonic irrigation once a week for four weeks.

As she continued on this program, Susan's sinus problems cleared up and her afternoon fatigue disappeared. In fact, she had often felt depressed but never associated the feeling of depression with her diet. Now, as the other symptoms disappeared, her depression also ended.

After about five weeks, the only remaining symptom was itchy skin. She decided to experiment. She began wearing clothing made exclusively of natural fibers—cotton, wool, rayon. Within 14 days, her skin condition, too, had healed; there was no more redness, no more itching.

## For Your Information

Here is a source of nonallergenic vitamins and supplements:

Freeda Vitamins      Dr. Philip Zimmerman
36 East 41 Street      Nutritional Hotline
New York, NY 10017      1-800-777-3737
(212) 685-4980

# 4

# Anemia

When your red-blood-cell count is too low, your body does not receive the oxygen it requires. As a result, you may show the typical symptoms of *anemia*—excessive fatigue, easy loss of breath, pallor—and your resistance to infections may be lowered.

Anemia may be the direct result of gastrointestinal bleeding, heavy menstruation, recurrent infections, or excessive breakdown of blood cells. In addition, anemia may be caused by a deficiency of a specific vitamin or mineral such as iron, copper, folic acid, vitamin $B_6$, and vitamin $B_{12}$.

Although anemia is commonly treated with iron supplements or vitamin $B_{12}$, the specific cause of the anemia must first be determined in order to treat each case properly.

## Folic Acid Deficiency Anemia

The most common cause of folic acid deficiency is poor diet, especially a diet lacking in dark-green, leafy vegetables. Because alcohol interferes with the metabolism of folic acid, alcohol abusers are especially susceptible to folic acid deficiency anemia. In addition, folic acid deficiency anemia may result from loss of blood (as from a tumor) and from celiac disease, a digestive disorder that upsets the body's ability to absorb nutrients. (See "Celiac Disease" on page 00).

Your body obtains folic acid from bacteria produced in your small intestine, as well as from foods and supplements. However, antacids and antibiotics can block the production and absorption of folic acid, especially (1) in older people and (2) when antacids and antibiotics are used in combination.

*Antacids.* Stomach acid is necessary for the absorption of folic acid. Because antacids slow down the stomach's secretion of acid, they may prevent proper absorption of folic acid.

*Antibiotics.* Antibiotics destroy intestinal bacteria. If you are taking both antacids and antibiotics (especially over a long period), your chances of becoming anemic are increased.

## Pernicious Anemia

Pernicious anemia is a very serious, possibly fatal disorder caused by a deficiency of vitamin $B_{12}$. In such cases, including vitamin $B_{12}$ in the diet and in supplements is not enough because there may be an inherited inability to absorb the vitamin $B_{12}$. Folic acid may conceal the symptoms of pernicious anemia. Therefore, folic acid supplements greater than 1.0 milligrams daily should be avoided.

Obviously, pernicious anemia requires the attention of a health care professional.

## Iron Deficiency Anemia

The American Academy of Pediatrics' Committee on Nutrition recommends *not* introducing cow's milk into an infant's diet too early in an effort to avoid iron deficiency anemia.

## Eat Foods Rich in Iron

Iron-rich foods are especially effective in combating anemia. Consider the following foods:

**Fruits**

| | |
|---|---|
| Apples | Plums |
| Apricots | Raisins |
| Bananas | Black currants |
| Dark grapes | Strawberries |

**Vegetables**

| | | |
|---|---|---|
| Alfalfa | Onions | Squash |
| Beets | Okra | Swiss chard |
| Broccoli | Potatoes | Tomatoes |
| Carrots | Radishes | Watercress |
| Kale | Spinach | Yams |

**Other Iron-Rich Foods**

Sunflower seeds

Black beans

Peas

Crude (unsulfured) blackstrap molasses

At the same time, be sure to avoid caffeinated beverages. Caffeine interferes with the body's ability to absorb iron. Also, increase your intake of protein.

## Use Supplements That Build Red Blood Cells

To regenerate red blood cells, be sure to include protein in your daily diet and to supplement your diet with the following vitamins and minerals: copper, iron, vitamin C, folic acid, vitamin $B_6$, and vitamin $B_{12}$.

Iron is retained and absorbed better when it is taken together with vitamin C.

## Juice Therapy

Enjoy any of the following freshly pressed vegetable and fruit juices:

### Vegetables

| | | |
|---|---|---|
| Alfalfa sprouts | Carrots | Swiss chard |
| Beets | Kale | Tomatoes |
| Broccoli | Spinach | Watercress |

### Fruits

| | |
|---|---|
| Apricots | Plums |
| Dark grapes | Strawberries |

For juice recipes that are especially helpful in fighting anemia, see Juice Therapy Formulas #8, 17, and 19 in the Appendix.

## Use Herbs to Your Advantage

In a controlled research study, Dr. K. Halwax of Australia found that the red-blood-cell count was much higher in patients who were given regular amounts of garlic extract over a period of eight weeks.

Try this herbal combination: comfrey root, raw garlic extract, dandelion, fenugreek kelp, and raspberry leaves.

## Aroma Therapy

Aroma therapy, too, can be useful in building red blood cells. For example, use chamomile, garlic, and lemon.

## Tissue Salts

Combine the following tissue salts:

Calcium phosphate
Ferrous phosphate
Potassium chloride
Sodium chloride
Sodium phosphate

# 5

# Arthritis

Arthritis is a joint disease which ranges from a mild, annoying condition to a severe, crippling disability. A very common ailment, arthritis is often incorrectly named as the cause for *any* pain in a joint or a bone.

## Types of Arthritis That Can Be Helped with Natural Therapies

*Rheumatoid Arthritis.* More common in women, rheumatoid arthritis generally appears between the ages of 25 and 50. Unlike the other types of arthritis, rheumatoid arthritis is considered a disease of the whole system, not simply of the joints.

*Infectious Arthritis.* This type of arthritis results directly from another disease (for example, from syphilis, gonorrhea, or tuberculosis) and usually settles in one joint.

*Osteoarthritis.* Generally associated with the elderly and the extremely overweight, osteoarthritis usually appears after the age of 40—often in a joint that has been previously injured.

*Gouty Arthritis.* Commonly known as *the gout*, this painful condition is caused by retention of uric acid in the tissues and the blood. Typically, the affected joint is the toe, which becomes red and swollen. Nutritional therapy is especially effective for this condition.

*Traumatic Arthritis.* A form of osteoarthritis, traumatic arthritis is always the result of a physical injury to a joint; for example, a blow, a strain, or wear and tear.

## Primary Causes of Arthritis

Many natural healers believe that arthritis is not a disease at all, but instead, a symptom of a deeper emotional/physical imbalance. Besides emotional stress and tension, the causes of arthritis include:

- Athletic injuries.
- Poor posture.
- Poor sleeping habits.
- Lack of exercise or imbalanced exercising.
- Nutritional stress from eating too fast and washing down unchewed foods with liquids.
- Low digestive enzyme activity, which results in poor assimilation of essential nutrients (especially minerals) and is often indicated by excess gas, bloating, constipation, and occasionally diarrhea. Medical doctors can test for low digestive enzyme activity with *gastric analysis by radiotelemetry.*

Good nutrition, consequently, plays a major role in overcoming the effects of arthritic conditions.

## Foods to Favor

Many foods are perfectly acceptable for arthritic patients, but certain foods have demonstrated special healing powers and therefore deserve close attention. Among these special foods are:

- Sea "vegetables"—that is, *seaweed*, such as dulse, hiziki, wakamae, and kelp. Seaweed provides an abundance of vitamins and minerals.
- Other macrobiotic foods—not only seaweed but also whole grains and beans.
- Cherries and cherry juice.
- Fresh fruit and vegetable juices.
- Raw potato juice.
- Parsley, alfalfa, watercress, string beans, wheat grass, and garlic.
- Wheat germ oil (one tablespoon a day).
- Blackstrap molasses—unsulfured (one tablespoon a day).

## Foods to Avoid

People who suffer from arthritis should pay special attention to the value of nutritional therapy. Here, for example, are some key foods to avoid:

| | |
|---|---|
| Refined breakfast cereals | Coffee and tea |
| Canned foods | White rice, white flour, |
| Roasted nuts and seeds | and white sugar |
| Anything with hydrogenated | Jams and jellies |
| fats or oils (Read the | Soft drinks |
| package labels carefully!) | Meats |
| Alcohol | |

Perhaps you're wondering why meats are on the above list. One of the world's most renowned nutrition researchers, Dr. Roger Williams, has found a connection between arthritis and atherosclerosis (hardening of the arteries). He suggests taking the same steps to avoid arthritis as you would take to avoid atherosclerosis, namely, avoid meats and high-cholesterol foods. The raw food or modified raw food diet described next is perfectly suitable.

## Use a Modified Raw Food Diet

Raw food diets have been very effective in helping patients lose extra weight, which contributes, of course, to joint pain in arthritics. To begin a modified raw food diet, follow these simple steps:

• Eliminate meat, fish, eggs, and poultry. You may do this gradually.

• As you eliminate flesh proteins, replace them with yogurt, buttermilk, or other fermented milk products. Use raw, certified goat's milk, if available.

• Eat numerous small meals rather than few large meals.

• Eat at least one large green salad each day.

• Eat at least one medium-size (six-ounce) fruit salad daily.

• Make a broth with cooked zucchini, string beans, turnips, and green leafy vegetables like watercress and parsley. This highly alkaline "potassium broth" helps reduce the acid intoxication of arthritis sufferers.

## Fasting for Pain-Free Results

Follow this step-by-step fasting program for relief from arthritis pains.

1. For about five days, limit your food intake to fresh fruits and vegetables.

2. During this five-day period, cleanse the colon by taking five to ten alfalfa tablets daily along with psyllium seed husks (one teaspoon of husks to eight ounces of water). Also, take bentonite, a volcanic ash that is available in most health food stores.

3. After five days, begin adding juices and the potassium broth made with cooked zucchini, string beans, turnips, and green leafy vegetables like watercress and parsley.

4. Continue this juice-and-broth fast for five to seven days. Note: Unless you are under the supervision of a qualified professional, do not undergo longer or stricter fasts.

5. To break the fast, eat fresh fruit or a blended salad. Mix green leafy vegetables with vegetable broth in an electric blender.

If your muscles ache while you are fasting, mix the following ingredients, then drink the mixture slowly:

1/2 tablespoon Alfalfa powder

1 tablespoon Unfiltered honey

1 tablespoon Apple cider vinegar

8 ounces Water

You will get rapid relief!

## Specific Dos and Don'ts

Follow these dos and don'ts for relief from specific types of arthritis pain.

### Gout

• Avoid foods high in purines, including organ meats, bouillon, gravy, yeast, and certain fish (particularly anchovies, herring, and sardines).

• Eat cherries (either fresh or frozen) or drink cherry juice. Cherries are especially strong in fighting the symptoms of gout.

• Lose weight, but do not begin your diet while you are suffering from an acute gout attack. Dieting will initially increase the uric acid in your blood.

**Rheumatoid Arthritis**

• Avoid chicken, fish, grains, liver, and potatoes.
• Remove fats and oils from your diet.
• Reduce your sodium intake to the minimum required.
• For pain relief, (1) follow a vegan diet (no meat, poultry, fish, dairy products, and eggs); (2) avoid coffee, tea, alcohol, and strong spices; and (3) supplement your vegan diet with vitamin $B_{12}$.
• Follow a raw food diet, but be sure to add fermented dairy products.
• Add to your diet the following fruits:

| | |
|---|---|
| Lemons | Grapefruits |
| Grapes | Apricots |
| Plums | Cherries |
| Black currants | Blackberries |

Also add to your diet these important greens: parsley, alfalfa, watercress, and string beans. In addition, add mung bean sprouts.

## Supplements That Provide Relief

Many respected researchers have reported positive results from a wide range of supplements. Not only vitamins and minerals but many other kinds of supplements contribute to the healing process, including special oils, enzymes, amino acids, and nutritional powders. In fact, research shows that combining certain supplements is especially beneficial. Therefore, be sure to take a high-potency multivitamin-mineral formula daily.

The following supplements are especially effective in healing arthritis pains. However, be sure to use supplements that are free of corn, wheat, soy, and yeast. Dr. Philip Zimmerman, a researcher on supplementation, and a respected scientist, reports that people who are sensitive to these items may have allergic reactions that mimic arthritis symptoms.

*Amino Acids.* L-Ornithine is a very effective remedy against arthritis. DL-Phenylalanine has a potent anti-inflammatory action for people suffering from osteoarthritis and rheumatoid arthritis.

*Zinc and Manganese.* Zinc helps reduce joint swelling and pain in certain kinds of arthritis. According to Dr. Carl Pfeiffer of the Brain BioCenter in Princeton, many arthritis sufferers have low levels of zinc and manganese and high levels of copper. For rheumatoid arthritis, he recommends daily supplementation with zinc, manganese, niacin, vitamin C, and two eggs (if you cannot eat eggs, substitute 200 milligrams of elemental sulfur).

*Free-Radical Scavengers.* Your body normally creates *free radicals*, chemical substances that may damage your synovial fluid (the fluid that lubricates the joints). Nutrients that are known to act as scavengers with free radicals are vitamins A, E, C, $B_1$, $B_5$, and $B_6$, as well as inositol and selenium. You may require high amounts of vitamins C (over 1,000 milligrams) and E (over 800 iu).

Certain types of arthritis result from problems involving the immune system. Nutrients that can trigger an immune response are the vitamins A, C, and E; the minerals selenium and zinc; and the amino acids arginine, ornithine, and cysteine.

*The B Vitamins.* To spur the natural healing process in the treatment of arthritis, be sure to take B vitamins. The B vitamins—especially when taken together with vitamin C—are powerful tools for healing joint inflammation and stiffness. High doses of vitamin $B_6$ (as much as 200 milligrams, three times a day) are very effective, especially for hand pain.

Vitamin $B_{12}$ injections (in doses of 30 to 900 mcg a week) can help reduce the side effects of cortisone, which medical doctors often administer to relieve inflammation in arthritics. At the same time, vitamin $B_{12}$ injections help alleviate poor assimilation or low digestive activity.

*PABA (Para-Aminobenzoic Acid).* Several holistic physicians claim that they have seen some cases in which PABA makes it possible to reduce the amount of cortisone needed to treat arthritis.

*Vitamin C, Pantothenic Acid, and Royal Jelly.* Vitamin C helps prevent the capillary walls in the joints from breaking down and causing swelling, bleeding, and pain. Vitamin C also relieves the back pain frequently associated with arthritis, according to Dr. James Greenwood, a Houston neurosurgeon.

Further, vitamin C and pantothenic acid help the adrenal glands to produce cortisone. After each meal, take one to three grams of buffered vitamin C and 50 to 100 milligrams of pantothenic acid.

*The Lancet,* the respected British journal of medicine, reports that pantothenic acid (administered by injection) and royal jelly, the food used to feed queen bees, has a positive effect in cases of rheumatoid arthritis.

*Vitamin E.* Vitamin E has anti-inflammatory properties that prove very helpful to arthritis sufferers. Also, arthritic patients often report that their fingers and toes feel cold. Vitamin E stimulates circulation, and in doses of 400 to 800 iu, it reduces muscular weakness, stiffness, and spasm.

*Propolis.* Propolis is a mixture of many nutrients and antibacterial agents. Gathered by bees, propolis is considered one of the most powerful natural healing agents.

*Calcium.* Calcium supplementation is essential for arthritis patients. Calcium helps relieve arthritis pain. In addition, calcium and vitamin C work together to form cartilage around the joints. Losing this cartilage is one cause of arthritis.

*Cod Liver Oil.* Spurned by many medical doctors as a "quack remedy," cod liver oil *does* help reduce the symptoms of arthritis, according to a study in the *Journal of the National Medical Association* (July 1959).

Begin by taking one-third teaspoon mixed in orange or grapefruit juice each day. If you wish, increase the amount to one tablespoon a day. Be sure to refrigerate the bottle and keep it tightly capped!

*Niacinamide.* Not to be confused with niacin, niacinamide has been proven very effective in reducing the pain of osteoarthritis and increasing joint mobility, especially in cases of degenerative arthritis of the knees. But while niacinamide controls the symptoms, it does not cure the disease. When the niacinamide treatment ends, the symptoms return.

Niacinamide is a type of vitamin $B_3$. For best results, take vitamins C and D along with niacinamide in the following recommended dosage:

1. 1,000 milligrams niacinamide (time-released formula) three times a day

2. 1,000 milligrams vitamin C (time-released, buffered, and with bioflavonoids) three times a day

3. 1,000 milligrams vitamin D

If you should become nauseous, reduce the dosage of niacinamide.

*Iron and Folic Acid.* Because many arthritis patients have anemia, treatments with iron, folic acid, and vitamin $B_{12}$ are very helpful.

*Betain Hydrochloride (Betain HCL).* If you have poor assimilation or low digestive activity, add betain hydrochloride to your list of supplements.

## Juice Therapy

Juice therapy is especially effective in treating the symptoms of arthritis. Always use freshly pressed juice, not canned or bottled juice.

See the Appendix for Juice Therapy Formula #8, 21, 22, 23 and 24.

If you suffer from gout, here is an especially helpful formula: Add four ounces of distilled water to twelve ounces of cherry juice. Drink this mixture for relief from gout pains.

Drink fresh pineapple juice. Many nutritional consultants believe that the enzyme bromelain, which is found in pineapples, reduces swelling and inflammation in different kinds of arthritis.

## Drink Herb Teas

Many different kinds of herbs have long been used in tea form to treat arthritis, including alfalfa, burdock, sage, and sassafras.

Herbalists believe that rosemary and comfrey contain a form of natural cortisone that reduces inflammation quickly. Indians used horsetail for its high silica content. They also used chaparral, which they gave the Spanish name *gobernadora*, "governor of the body."

## Apply Herb Oils and Salves

Over the centuries, the most popular use of herbs in the treatment of arthritis has been in topical form. Oils and salves have been very effective in soothing inflamed and swollen joints.

Precisely why herb salves work so effectively is still unclear. Perhaps as the oils are absorbed through the skin, the herbs increase the supply of blood to the affected muscle or joint by reflex action. In any case, the most effective herb salves generally contain one or more of the following: camphor, cayenne pepper (capsicum), clove oil, menthol, methyl salicylate, thymol, turpentine oil.

Compresses of flaxseed, mustard plasters, and paraffin wax have also been popular for many years.

Try these special herbal salves for relief from arthritis pain:

• Rub a smooth layer of castor oil on the skin. On this first layer, place a layer of Tiger Balm or Olbas Oil (both are commercially made salves). The castor oil has a healing quality all its own. Moreover, it prevents blistering and chafing from other, more irritating oils.

• When one of your joints flares up from arthritis, apply a mixture of wheat germ oil and wintergreen, then wrap the area with a moist, warm towel. To keep the warmth in, wrap the towel with wool or cotton flannel.

• For a most effective salve, mix the following ingredients:

| | |
|---|---|
| 1/4 teaspoon wheat germ oil | 1/4 teaspoon cajuput oil |
| 1 teaspoon wintergreen oil | 1 teaspoon cayenne pepper |
| 1/4 teaspoon mustard oil | 4 teaspoons castor oil |
| 1/4 teaspoon rosemary oil | 3 ounces gum camphor |

For pain relief, apply the mixture to the affected area and wrap the area with flannel.

## Aroma Therapy

The general essences used to soothe the pains of arthritic conditions are garlic, juniper, lemon, onion, and thyme. If you suffer from gout or rheumatoid arthritis, these specific essences may be especially helpful in aroma therapy:

*Gout:* essence of garlic, juniper, rosemary, basil, cajuput, fennel, lemon, pine, thyme.

*Rheumatoid Arthritis:* Essence of German chamomile (contains azulene, which is especially effective against the bacterial agent present in acute rheumatoid arthritis), eucalyptus, garlic, juniper, lemon, origanum, terebinth, and thyme.

## Massage Away Stiffness and Pain

Massage is most useful when you experience stiffness and pain without swelling or inflammation. The two most powerful techniques for massaging arthritic joints are (1) circular rhythmic pressure and (2) kneading, both of which are described in the Appendix.

## Be Sure to Exercise!

Exercise is essential for everyone, and it is especially beneficial if you have arthritis. It provides movement and flexibility, without which your muscles become stiff and stagnant.

## Range-of-Motion Exercises

Range-of-motion exercises help you evaluate just how well you can move your muscles and joints. At the same time, of course, they also improve flexibility of the joints, even joints affected by arthritis. By fully rotating each joint, you will relieve tightness in the area.

Here is a wonderful range-of-motion exercise you might try to help all areas of your body.

• Stand tall, even if you feel somewhat stiff. Now slowly and gently begin to rotate the joints in the upper part of the body: first your jaw; then your neck and shoulders; next your elbows; finally, your wrist and fingers.

Put each joint through its complete range of motion; that is, move it in every normal way the joint should move. Do not force movement if you feel stiffness and discomfort.

• Next, lie back on a soft cushion. If you are uncomfortable on your back, then use an arm chair. Slowly begin to rotate your legs in a bicycling motion. This movement will loosen your hips and knees. Now rotate your ankles and move your toes.

To exercise your fingers, try crumpling a newspaper and squeezing it tightly. If you prefer, use a rubber ball instead. Either exercise will help keep your finger and hand muscles strong and pliable.

## Tai Chi and Hatha Yoga

Ready for advanced exercising? Try tai chi or hatha yoga!

These forms of exercise are among the best for arthritis sufferers, because they place little stress on joints and are easy to perform. Consult your yellow pages for a local exercise center, a "Y," or an adult education program that offers tai chi or yoga classes.

## A Word of Warning About Exercising

If a joint becomes very swollen or inflamed, you should try only the lightest, least strenuous exercises or avoid exercising altogether while the joint is in this condition. If a joint becomes stiff or sore from 6 to 12 hours after you exercise, reduce the amount of exercise.

## Hydrotherapy and Other Techniques

Hydrotherapy and a number of miscellaneous techniques have proved helpful in cases of arthritis.

*Ice Packs.* Studies have shown that applying ice packs to the knees of arthritic people reduces pain and increases mobility.

*Fangotherapy.* In this treatment, which is used at the Moriah Dead Sea Spa Hotel in Israel, heated sea mud is applied to arthritic joints. Fangotherapy is also used for rehabilitation after a fracture.

*Bath Oils.* For arthritis and rheumatism, try juniper oil baths. Also, try oil baths with marjoram, thyme, rosemary, or sage. For affected (but not inflamed) joints, try warm castor oil compresses, covered with a heating pad.

*Heat Therapy.* Applying moist heat is often the most effective way to treat pain. Try this mixture. Dissolve the following ingredients in a pint of water: one ounce Epsom salts, one teaspoon table salt, one teaspoon bicarbonate of soda.

Take a square piece of wool or cotton flannel and soak this fabric in the salt solution. Place the soaked material on the affected area. Cover the compress with a thick piece of cloth to retain the heat. Avoid using heat, however, when you have pain, swelling and inflammation at the same time.

*Enemas.* Taking an enema once or twice a week often helps relieve arthritis symptoms.

*Showers.* Alternating hot and cold showers, together with dry brushing, may stimulate the adrenal and other glands to create cortisone, a natural healer. Proceed as follows:

Begin with a 10- to 15-minute shower of very warm water—never hot enough to cause discomfort. Then switch to three minutes of cool water. Alternate this procedure three or four times, always finishing with a cool shower. Use a firm brush or a terry cloth towel to give your body a "dry brush" massage.

## Homeopathy

Consider the following specific homeopathy techniques:

- For arthritis pain—salix nig.
- For joint pain—coffea.
- For rheumatic pain, swollen joints, and arthritis pain—rhus tox.
- For rheumatic pain—cimicifuga or apis.

Tissue salts can be very helpful for arthritis pains:

- For soothing sore joints—silica and magnesium phosphate.
- For reducing inflammation—iron phosphate.
- For chronic complaints—sodium phosphate, sodium chloride (not common table salt!), and silica.
- For damaged tissues—silicea and calcium fluoride (in 30X potency). The damaged tissues may be able to absorb these high-potency remedies and help the cells regain some elasticity and strength.

The Natra Bio Company makes a homeopathic product specifically for the pain, swollen joints, stiff limbs, and other symptoms associated with arthritis. The formula is called #508 and contains:

| | |
|---|---|
| Salix nig., 4X | Bryonia, 6X |
| Coffea, 3X | Cimicifuga, 4X |
| Rhus. tox., 6X | Apis, 9X |

For further information, contact:

Natra Bio Company
506 Santa Monica Blvd.
Santa Monica, CA 90401

## Edgar Cayce Remedies

The oils and oil combinations that were often mentioned in the Cayce readings for arthritis are: peanut oil, olive oil, oil of pine needles, and sassafras oil.

You might add to these wintergreen and cedarwood oil.

## The Value of Rest and Relaxation

In the *natural* healing process, rest and relaxation are two potent natural tools! Keeping yourself as emotionally calm and stress-free as possible helps enable your body's healing powers to take effect. When you are suffering from stiff, inflamed tissues, resting will be especially helpful.

Generally speaking, the more effectively you can rest, the faster the healing process can be completed. Therefore, you really should learn to rest.

- Take three or four 20-minute naps during the day.
- Try using a water bed to improve your sleeping posture. Improper posture while you are asleep can cut off the oxygen supply to a certain part of your body, say, to a joint. Over a period of time, repeatedly sleeping in the same position will make the joint stiff and deformed.
- If you wake up with backaches, check your mattress. If it is sagging, replace it with a new, firm mattress. Or place a sheet of plywood (about one-half inch thick) between your mattress and the bed springs for improved support.
- Using a sleeping bag may help avoid that early morning stiffness. Why? Because a sleeping bag helps keep your body temperature uniform. For this reason, sleeping bags are more effective than heating pads.
- Do you wake up with stiff hands? Use a pair of stretch gloves for greater hand flexibility. Be sure that the gloves are not too tight and do not cut off circulation.
- Check that your pillow is not too high. A pillow that raises your head too high may be harmful for arthritis patients.
- If you have arthritis in the hips or knees, do not sleep with a pillow under your knees. Instead, try to sleep flat on your back, with all your joints straight, but not rigid. If you keep a joint bent and inactive over a period of time, the inactive muscles will contract around the affected joint and cause more pain.

## Control Pain Through Visualization Techniques

Try using visualization to control the pain of arthritis. Visual imagery helps reduce tension, alleviate stress, and relieve pain. Just close your eyes, get into a relaxed position, and begin. Here is a step-by-step visualization technique that arthritis sufferers may find especially helpful for controlling pain.

Find a quiet place where you will not be disturbed. Sit in a straight-back chair with both feet flat on the floor. Rest your hands palms up on your knees. Close your eyes. Inhale and exhale long and slowly. Breathe deeply, slowly, and rhythmically. As you do so, visualize the area or part of your body where the pain is centered. As you inhale, visualize a blue light entering your body. With each breath you take, the blue light enters your body, surrounds the painful area, and soothes the pain. Focus intensely on this blue energy that is entering your body and dissolving the pain. As you exhale, visualize clearly how the pain is leaving your body in the form of a gray cloud. Continue with this exercise until you feel relief and a sense of relaxation. To finish, take a long, deep breath, slowly exhale, and gradually open your eyes. Remain seated and stay quiet for a few minutes as you become aware once again of your surroundings. Slowly begin to wiggle your toes and fingers. Rise whenever you feel you are ready.

## Also of Interest

You will find the following miscellaneous notes interesting and helpful:

- Food allergies frequently cause the symptoms of arthritis. Of course, the best "cure" is to avoid the foods that bother you. Vitamin $B_{12}$ injections and digestive enzyme supplements may be helpful, but most other nutritional supplements are of limited value.

• Beware of dietary programs that promise an "arthritis cure." Many of these programs instruct you to avoid certain foods—for example, citrus fruits—that supposedly cause acid intoxication, which in turn, further aggravates arthritis symptoms. Certain arthritis sufferers may indeed have a sensitivity to citrus fruits. However, oranges and other citrus fruits are known to have an *alkaline* effect on the system and in certain situations may actually assist in the healing process.

• Prescription drugs may have side effects that resemble arthritis symptoms. Arthritis and hypertension are both associated with high levels of stress, and many people with high blood pressure take thiazide drugs. One side effect of drugs in the thiazide family is elevation of the level of uric acid in the blood, and uric acid contributes to certain arthritic symptoms.

• One popular folk remedy is to melt paraffin wax and paint it onto arthritic joints.

• Heat helps alleviate arthritis pain. An infrared lamp is the most effective method of producing heat. Ultrasound therapy produces deep, internal heat.

• When your joints are swollen and inflamed, intense heat, deep massage, and exercise will aggravate the symptoms. Instead, rest and put cool packs on the inflamed area.

• Instead of artificial light, use natural light and full-spectrum lamps whenever possible in home and office.

• If you have low stomach acid, you can aid your digestion by mixing two teaspoons of apple cider vinegar in a glass of water and drinking the mixture before or with your meals.

• The test that doctors use to diagnose arthritis is called ESR, *e*rythrocyte *s*edimentation *r*ate. This test measures the rate at which red blood cells, erythrocytes, settle to the bottom of a glass tube.

• In their book *Life Extension*, Durk Pearson and Sandy Shaw explain that complexes of aspirin and copper (copper salicylates) have enzyme properties that may reduce inflammation. Perhaps this information sheds some light on the old folk remedy about wearing copper bracelets to reduce arthritis pain.

• TNS therapy has been found effective in reducing the pain of rheumatoid arthritis. TNS (*t*ranscutaneous *n*erve *s*timulator) therapy is a technique that involves the use of various degrees of electrical stimulation to help reduce pain. It has been found to be most helpful for musculoskeletal pain of the neck, shoulders, and back.

## How Dorothy H. Found Relief From Osteoarthritis

Dorothy H. had osteoarthritis. She greatly damaged her health by eating highly processed foods and drinking two to three cups of coffee a day, and she was under great stress. Dorothy had troubles with her stomach and bowels, she had trouble sleeping, and her swollen joints constantly ached.

At first, she made a half-hearted effort. She stopped drinking coffee and began exercising. But this wasn't enough. Finally, she made a full commitment to regaining her health. She began a one-week fast of alkaline broth and vegetable juices. By the fourth day, she noticed a marked difference: her joints were less stiff and less red than before. At the same time, she began using visualization techniques. After her fast,

Dorothy started a modified raw food diet. When she started her diet, Dorothy also began swimming regularly—slowly at first, gradually increasing the number of laps.

Only 30 days after she had begun her new health program, Dorothy had total relief from her arthritis symptoms. Now, she experiences her old daily symptoms rarely—only during extreme climate changes or when she goes off her program.

## For Your Information

Here is an all-volunteer, nonprofit organization that designs and manufactures devices for handicapped people, whether the cause of the handicap is arthritis or some other ailment:

The Independence Factory
P. O. Box 597
Middletown, Ohio 45042

# 6

## Bladder Disorders

The most common disorders of the bladder include:

- Bladder and Urethra irritation
- Bladder infection (cystitis)
- Bladder problems due to food allergies
- Bladder stones (these form in the bladder or enter the bladder from the kidney).

### Nutritional Considerations

- Fasting for a few (two to three) days is very valuable in accelerating the healing of bladder infections.
- Modified raw food diet (see Appendix). Emphasis on nuts and whole grains.
- Some people are sensitive to the fluorine and chlorine in tap water and react to them. For this reason distilled water is the best choice of drinking water in the healing of any bladder disorder.
- It is valuable to use foods high in lactobacillus acidophilus such as homemade yogurt and buttermilk.
- Take one tablespoon of apple cider vinegar in eight ounces of distilled water each morning until the burning upon urination passes. Then continue using this combination for five more days.

## Juice Therapy

• Juice Therapy Formula #6. Add a small amount of onion or garlic to this formula.

• Drink 8 ounces of cranberry juice three times per day. This will acidify the urine and reduce bacterial activity that may be causing the bladder infections.

• Watermelon juice.

## Herbs for Bladder Disorders

Yarrow, witch hazel, juniper berries, goldenseal, uva ursi, buchu, cleavers.

Cystitis—Echinacea extract. Five to ten drops every hour.

## Hydrotherapy for Cystitis

1. Hot herbal compresses.

2. Hot sitz baths (98 - 99 degrees F.) for one-half hour, twice daily. Add water to keep temperature constant. This is not recommended for someone with heart trouble.

3. Warm catnip tea taken in an enema (one tablespoon dried catnip to a quart of water).

## Homeopathy

• Cystitis—Urtica (nettles)

• Bladder irritability, incontenance, frequent and difficult urination with pain—Triticum.

• Desire for frequent urination, difficult and scanty urination—Thiaspi, Terebinthina

• Bladder irritation—Buchu.

## Tissue Salts Recommended

• Bladder irritation—Ferr. Phos.

## Miscellaneous Notes of Interest

A RAST test is recommended if the condition does not respond to the measures described above. This test will determine if food allergies may be at the root of the disorder.

# 7

# Cancer

Perhaps no other disease receives as much attention today as cancer. Actually, cancer is not one disease but over 100 different diseases that share a common problem: the uncontrolled growth and spread of abnormal cells.

No one who has cancer should attempt self-treatment. Anyone who has—or suspects that he or she might have—cancer should consult a health professional.

Precisely how effective specific natural healing techniques are in cancer cases is the subject of much controversy, and the dispute will probably continue for years to come. On the one hand, natural healers report success in dealing with cancer in some cases. On the other hand, medical and government organizations claim that so-called "natural treatments" are simply obstacles preventing patients from receiving valuable help.

There is evidence, however, that most cancers *are* caused by controllable factors. Dr. Marvin A. Schneiderman, Chief Statistician of the National Cancer Institute, said that the number of cancer cases could be very drastically cut if people would change their lifestyles. [Judith Randall, "Help Yourself to Stave Off Cancer," *New York Daily News*, March 31, 1976.]

Although most cancers are caused by controllable factors, we can make no guaranty or claim, even when we have substantial evidence. There are far too many factors involved. Simply put, the subject of cancer is as complicated as it is controversial!

## Causes of Cancer

Since "cancer" is really over 100 different diseases, there could possibly be over 100 different causes. The causes that have been most closely associated with cancer are:

- Excessive exposure to the sun
- Certain chemicals found in our air and our water
- Certain food additives and cosmetic additives
- Viral infections
- Ionizing radiation
- Vitamin and mineral deficiencies
- Negative emotions in certain types of cancer
- Aflatoxins in peanuts
- Excessive use of dietary fats
- Carcinogens found in meats

## Common Warning Signs

Spotting one or more of the common symptoms of cancer does not necessarily "prove" anything. Many cancer symptoms are also symptoms of other, less serious disorders. In any case, before you jump to conclusions, discuss all your symptoms with a knowledgeable physician, one who will take the time to evaluate among other things, your lifestyle, your emotional and family history, and your eating and exercise habits.

The most common warning signs are:

- Change in bladder or bowel patterns
- Chronic cough or hoarseness
- Constant indigestion
- Difficulty in swallowing
- Thickening of tissue anywhere on the body (especially on the breast)
- Major change in a mole or a wart
- A sore that refuses to heal
- An unusual discharge
- Unusual bleeding

In addition, there are a number of less common warning signs.

- Unusual and chronic headaches accompanied by unusual behavior and changes in visual perception
- Chronic fatigue
- Chronic low-grade fever
- Constant pain in the bones with no apparent cause
- Excessive bruising of the skin
- Loss of appetite, unusual weight loss, or both.

Again, be sure not to reach any conclusions based simply on your observation of what might be one or more of the common signs. *Always* consult a health professional.

## Natural Healing and Cancer

Clearly, discussing *all* the issues and therapies surrounding this complicated subject is beyond the scope of this book. Therefore, we will focus on the most effective natural approaches for reducing the chances of getting cancer.

Despite all the different opinions, different approaches, and different theories, most natural healers generally agree with these three broad ways to prevent cancer:

- Reduce or eliminate animal protein from your diet.
- Eliminate all carcinogenic factors or influences in your life.
- Stimulate and detoxify your liver.

Further, natural healers agree that once a patient has cancer, it is important to address the emotional issues that may be involved in creating the breakdown that has led to cancer.

## Preventing Cancer—The Basic Steps

Most intelligent people like you want to know, "What can I do to help prevent cancer?" Here are a few tips:

- Give up smoking.
- Give up alcohol.
- Follow a cancer-prevention food program.
- Limit your exposure to radiation. Use a protective shield during dental X rays. Unless absolutely necessary, avoid diagnostic X rays (such as mammographies).
- Avoid excessive exposure to the sun. Use a sunscreen whenever possible.
- Always follow safety regulations strictly, if your job places you in contact with any carcinogens.

## Natural Ways to Minimize Radiation Damage

The effects of radiation can include vomiting, diarrhea, hemorrhaging, and severe anemia. Studies have shown that these effects can be largely prevented by taking generous amounts of certain vitamins and supplements beginning several days *before* the radiation treatment.

*Vitamins B and C.* Along with vitamin C, take rutin and bioflavonoids to strengthen the capillaries and reduce hemorrhaging. Take pyridoxine (vitamin $B_6$) to prevent vomiting.

*Brewer's Yeast.* At Montefiore Hospital in New York, a study of two groups of patients scheduled to undergo heavy radiation was very interesting. One group was given brewer's yeast (or primary grown yeast); the other group was not. The patients who took three tablespoons daily of yeast beginning one week before treatment were symptom-free after treatment. Patients who did not take yeast suffered severe anemia and experienced vomiting.

*Other Helpful Nutrients.* You can reduce radiation damage by taking 50 milligrams of pantothenic acid daily prior to exposure. Yogurt also helps to neutralize radioactive chemicals in the intestines. In addition, the following supplements are known to be helpful: *glutathione, pectin, inositol, essential fatty acids, algin, lecithin, bee pollen,* and *lemon or lemon peel extract.*

## Adopt a Cancer-Prevention Food Program

Take a solid step toward preventing the incidence of cancer by following a carefully planned food program. Here are some recommendations.

- Increase your intake of cruciferous vegetables (cabbage and cauliflower, for example), whole grains, beans, and high-carotene foods such as carrots, collard greens, spinach, cantaloupe, beet greens, broccoli, apricots, papaya, prunes, peaches, watermelon, and squash (yellow, zucchini, butternut, acorn, and hubbard).

- Include strawberries and tomatoes in your diet. A low intake of both these foods has been associated with an increased risk of cancer.

- Take four tablespoons of pureed asparagus daily.

- Be sure to eat beans. Beans contain a protease inhibitor, which may block cancer.

- Reduce the amount of fat in your diet to no more than 20 percent of your total caloric intake. To do so, avoid or drastically cut your intake of vegetable oil, margarine, meat, and poultry. If you do eat poultry, remove the skin. Also, cut your intake of high-fat dairy products which include whole milk, sour cream, butter, cream cheese and other cheeses.

- Reduce your protein intake to between 12 and 18 percent of your diet.

- Avoid refined sugars whenever possible.

- Increase your intake of high-fiber foods.

- Increase your intake of foods high in vitamin A, vitamin C, vitamin E, vitamin B complex, and selenium.

- Eat more fresh fruits and vegetables, especially dark-green and deep-yellow vegetables.

- Do not eat foods that have been smoked, pickled, or barbecued. They contain carcinogens.

- Avoid any foods that contain nitrates and nitrites, additives commonly found in deli meats, bacon, and smoked fish, for example. These additives react with the body's amines to form nitrosamine compounds, which may cause cancer. If you do eat these foods occasionally increase your intake of vitamin C. Vitamin C interferes with the formation of nitrosamines.

- Avoid frying or broiling meats. The process of frying or broiling produces at least eight chemical mutagens that might contribute to certain types of cancer. Instead, learn how to steam, boil, bake, pressure-cook, stew, and poach your foods.

- Use stainless steel cookware. Do not use copper or aluminum cookware.

- Add foods rich in vitamins A and C to your diet.

- Drink distilled water. If you must drink chlorinated tap water, boil the water first. Avoid fluoridated water. Researchers have linked an increased cancer rate in certain cities to the presence of fluoridated water there.

- Increase your intake of dietary fiber, particularly whole grains, beans, fruits, and vegetables. Women with breast cancer have been found to excrete less *ligna*, a substance that is formed in higher amounts in fiber-rich diets and that probably plays a protective role.

- Avoid alcohol. Men who drink beer heavily may be predisposed to cancer of the rectum and bowels. Women who drink alcoholic beverages have a higher chance of developing breast cancer.

Some of these recommendations are loosely based on Dr. Oliver Alabaster's *What You Can Do to Prevent Cancer* (Simon and Schuster, 1985).

## The Link Between Specific Types of Cancer and Diet

Let's focus on some specific types of cancer:

*Bladder Cancer.* In one study, women who drank coffee were 2½ times more likely to contract bladder cancer than women who did not drink coffee. Vitamin C may inhibit spontaneous tumor formation in the bladder.

*Breast Cancer and Uterine Cancer.* Obesity as well as a high intake of animal fats, cholesterol, and protein may contribute to breast and uterine cancer.

*Colon Cancer.* Meat and meat fat contribute to colon cancer.

*Stomach Cancer.* Pickled vegetables and smoked fish have been associated with stomach cancer. In one study, Japanese people whose diets were rich in these foods had higher rates of stomach cancer.

*Liver Cancer.* Excessive intake of vitamin A over a long period of time, alcohol, and a steady high-fat diet may contribute to liver cancer.

*Esophageal Cancer.* Combined heavy intake of tobacco smoke and alcohol contribute to this cancer.

*Rectal and Bowel Cancer.* Very heavy beer drinking may predispose men to rectal and bowel cancer, according to studies conducted by France's International Agency for Research on Cancer.

*Lung Cancer.* Tobacco use, of course, is associated with lung cancer. Also, people with a low beta carotene intake have a higher rate of lung cancer. The best food sources for carotene are

| | | |
|---|---|---|
| Apricots | Oranges | Sweet potatoes |
| Broccoli | Peaches | Sweet red peppers |
| Carrots | Tomatoes | Winter squash |
| Kale | Spinach | |

*Prostate Cancer.* A low-fat diet lessens the chances of cancer of the prostate. In one study, Japanese men who ate green and yellow vegetables had a lower rate of prostate cancer.

## Should You Become a Vegetarian?

In virtually all cultures, people who eat low-fiber, high-fat, high-meat diets have a greater risk of prostate, colon, and breast cancer.

On the other hand, a number of studies indicate that vegetarians have lower rates of certain types of cancer. Unlike meats, vegetables are not known to cause cancer; moreover, certain vegetables may actually *reduce* the risk of cancer.

Vegetables, whole grains, and beans contain vitamins A and C and dietary fiber, all of which may have cancer-blocking properties. In particular, vegetables of the mustard family (known as "cruciferous" vegetables because the four leaves surrounding their flowers suggest a cross) may reduce the risk of gastrointestinal cancer and respiratory cancer. Cruciferous vegetables, which include cabbage, cauliflower, brussels sprouts, kohlrabi, and broccoli, may also be very effective in protecting against chemically induced cancers.

"Vegetarian women excrete more estrogen and have less of this cancer-promoting hormone in their blood than meat-eating women," according to one study. [Jane E. Brody, "New Research on the Vegetarian Diet," *New York Times*, October 12, 1983, Section C, p. 8.]

All these factors weigh heavily in favor of adopting vegetarian dietary habits.

## Supplements Which May Contribute to Cancer Prevention

Admittedly, there have been too few controlled studies on the benefits of supplementation as a means of cancer prevention. However, research has shown that certain nutrients may act as preventives.

*Vitamins C and A.* Vitamin C may help protect against stomach cancer. Vitamin C may also help women who are susceptible to cervical cancer, and vitamin A may help men against prostate cancer. In large doses, vitamins C and A inhibit *hyaluronidase*, an enzyme found in cancerous tissues.

*Selenium and Vitamin E.* Selenium appears to prevent cancer by increasing the immune response. When used together, selenium and vitamin E increase antibody production and can be used in breast cancer treatment. They also act as antioxidants to reduce free-radical formation.

*Acidophilus.* Some acidophilus cultures retard the growth of cancer cells.

*Molybdenum.* A deficiency of molybdenum may be linked to cancer of the digestive tract.

*Bee Pollen.* Preliminary studies indicate that breast tumors may be prevented or delayed when bee pollen is added to food (1 part in 10,000). Studies showed that even existing tumors were reduced in size.

## Juices

You already know the general value of fresh vegetable and fruit juices. For a patient who is not too weak, a fast of raw fruits and vegetables may be helpful, but the fast should be short, say, only two or three days long.

In Europe, many naturopathic physicians recommend Biota Brand beet juice, which is available in many American health food stores.

In addition, try these juices:

• Mix the juice from carrots, spinach, and beets.
• Drink the juice of beet crystals.
• Mix carrot juice with black cherry juice.

Remember to use only *fresh* products for your juices.

## Herbal Remedies

Use the following herbs as cancer preventives: Jason Winters brand herbal tea (available in health food stores), asparagus puree, chaparral tea, red clover blossoms, dandelion root, Irish moss, and garlic.

## Does Your Emotional Health Play a Part?

Traditionally, cancer is not considered psychosomatic, that is, caused by mental or emotional disturbance. However, evidence that links our emotions with both the response of the immune system and the progress of a disease such as cancer is accumulating.

In the 1950s, the psychotherapist Lawrence LeShan sketched the first detailed profile of the "cancer-prone individual" as someone who suffers from feelings of desertion, loneliness, guilt, and self-condemnation. ["Are Cancer and Personality Linked?" *National Observer*, April 3, 1978, p. 1.] Subsequent studies have also linked emotions and feelings with our immune response, or more directly, with cancer.

• Breast cancer patients who showed strong motivation toward fighting their disease exhibit a stronger immune response and are, therefore, more likely to survive than patients who are "resigned to their fate."

• "Emotions such as anxiety, apathy, and depression may have a significant effect on immune system factors such as the natural killer cells that fight cancer. The studies point to links between the emotions and such diseases as flu, colds, and genital herpes, in addition to cancer." [Daniel Goldman, "Strong Emotional Response to Disease May Bolster Patient's Immune System," *New York Times*, October 22, 1985, Section C, page 1.]

• Cancer patients repress unpleasant feelings (depression, hostility, and guilt) to an abnormal degree. They may view their fathers as unprotective and nondemanding and their mothers as unloving, unrewarding, and unprotecting. ["Are Cancer and Personality Linked?" *National Observer*, April 3, 1978, p. 1.]

• Injury to certain parts of the brain have been shown to diminish immune function.

• Cancer patients who have the greatest chance of survival are those who take an active part in their own recovery.

Many researchers now acknowledge that the emotions are probably involved in the complicated chain of events that leads to a disease, most likely in the advanced stages of the illness.

## Visualization and Hypnosis

Hypnotized cancer patients have been trained to visualize their white blood cells overwhelming and devouring their cancer cells. The result? There has been visible improvement in their conditions using this approach.

## Heat Therapy

Heat has been used in various ways to treat cancer. For example, heat has been used to shrink cancerous tumors. In some studies, patients were anesthetized and their bodies were heated to 108 degrees by means of heated gas in the lungs and heated water blankets. Another approach uses the heat of radiofrequency radiation.

## Music Therapy

Music is helpful in reducing pain and emotional stress in cancer patients.

## For Your Information

Here are some sources that may interest you:

For more information on the effect of the emotions and visualization techniques on cancer:

Cancer Counseling & Research Center
1300 Summit Avenue, Suite 710
Fort Worth, Texas 76102

For information on the use of bacterial products in the treatment of cancer:

Helen Coley Nauts
Executive Director
Cancer Research Institute, Inc.
1225 Park Avenue
New York, NY 10128

For nutritional and holistic approaches to cancer therapy:

Linus Pauling Institute of Science
   and Medicine (1)
2700 Sand Hill Road
Menlo Park, CA 94025
(415) 854-0843

International Association of
   Cancer Victims and Friends
7740 West Manchester, Suite 110
Playa del Rey, CA 90291
(213) 822-5032

Cancer Control Society
2043 North Berendo
Los Angeles, CA 90027
(213) 663-7801

Project CURE (3)
2020 K Street, N.W., Suite 350
Washington, DC 20070
(202) 293-3479

Gerson Institute (2)
P.O. Box 430
Bonita, CA 92002
(619) 267-1150

The Arlin J. Brown Information
   Center
P.O. Box 251
Fort Belvoir, VA 22060

For products for women who have had mastectomies:

Natural Look Inc.
195 Mamaroneck Avenue
White Plains, NY 10602

(1)   Conducts research on vitamin C as a cancer treatment.
(2)   A nonprofit center for education and research.
(3)   A clearinghouse for alternative cancer therapies, Project CURE is operated by former cancer patients.

# 8

# Candida
# Albicans

As many as 80 million people may suffer from disorders caused by *Candida albicans*, a yeast that lives in all our bodies. Normal levels of the yeast cause no problems, but when abnormal growth pushes the level of *Candida albicans* higher, disorders can result; for example, oral thrush in children and vaginitis in women.

When the growth is unchallenged, the result can be a much more serious disease in which the yeast becomes a fungus that releases harmful toxins. Because these toxins weaken the immune system, they can in turn cause abdominal pain, allergies, bronchial problems, constipation, depression, diarrhea, headaches, irritability, memory loss, menstrual disorders, and skin disorders.

## What Causes the Problem?

*Candida albicans* can be caused by a number of different sources:

• Broad-spectrum antibiotics can destroy beneficial bacteria in the intestines. The beneficial bacteria are then replaced by *Candida albicans*.

• Stress, pollution, cortisone (and other steroid derivatives), and birth control pills can weaken the body's immune system and allow the *Candida albicans* to grow.

• Changes in normal gastrointestinal acidity.

• Chemotherapy to treat cancer.

• Repeated pregnancies.

• Poor nutrition, especially high-carbohydrate and high-meat diets. Meat-eaters are more susceptible to *Candida albicans* because they may ingest low levels of antibiotics normally fed to livestock.

## How Can It Be Cured?

Natural healers and holistic doctors believe that *Candida albicans* can be cured by: killing the yeast; cleansing the dead cells from the body; reestablishing normal digestive functions and an efficient metabolism; tonifying afflicted organs and glands; and reestablishing healthful colonies of the essential microorganisms in the body, including acidophilus, bulgaricus, and bifidus.

## Foods to Avoid and Foods to Favor

The most effective nutritional program to combat *Candida albicans* is a yeast-free, low-carbohydrate diet. Avoid baker's yeast and any baked goods that might contain it and brewer's yeast and any products that might contain it (for example, alcoholic beverages).

Also be sure to avoid refined sugars, vinegar, relishes, mushrooms, aged cheeses, dried fruits, and fruit juices.

Eat plenty of fresh vegetables, sea vegetables, grains, beans, and a small amount of fresh fruit.

## Herbal Remedies

Candida Cleanse is an herbal product specifically formulated to relieve *Candida albicans*. To obtain this product, contact

> Light Nutritional Systems
> P.O. Box 3033
> Santa Cruz, CA 95063
> (408) 429-9089 or 1-800-635-1233

Herbs that can be beneficial in a program to combat *Candida albicans* include black walnut, Pau D'Arco, echinacea, astragalus, fennel seed, marsh mallow root, horsetail, nettles, gentian, bladder wrack, Oregon grape root, chaparral, garlic, and thuja.

## Add Acidophilus to Your Diet

Acidophilus has a beneficial effect on *Candida albicans*. Also be sure to include in your diet any of the supplements that reduce stress and build the immune system, especially biotin and vitamin $B_{12}$. For thrush, take a B-complex vitamin along with acidophilus.

# 9

## Cardiovascular Disease

Natural healing is especially useful in preventing and treating cardiovascular disease—that is, disorders associated with the heart and the circulatory system. There are many different kinds of disorders in the family of cardiovascular diseases. Some are not very serious; others can cause disability and death. If you are determined to change your lifestyle, you can indeed address even the most serious cardiovascular conditions productively.

### Common Conditions

Various conditions belong to the cardiovascular family, the most common of which are:

*Atherosclerosis and Arteriosclerosis.* The names themselves are telling: *atheromas* are fat deposits, and *sclerosis* means "hardening." The fat deposits cause a thickening and hardening of the arteries that lead to such symptoms as hypertension, muscle cramping and paralysis, a feeling of heaviness in the chest area, and pains radiating from the chest into the left arm and left shoulder.

*Angina Pectoris.* Often simply called "angina," this disease causes pain around the heart, an indication of blocked or poor circulation. These symptoms generally appear after a period of emotional stress or physical exertion.

*Hypertension.* High blood pressure.

*Cardiac Arrhythmias.* Irregular heartbeats.

*Congestive Heart Failure.* The heart can be weakened as a result of beriberi, heart attack, rheumatic fever, arteriosclerosis, and hypothyroidism.

When the heart is weakened, it may not pump blood and other tissue fluids efficiently. As a result of this poor circulation, fluid may back up into the lungs and other organs. The symptoms of congestive heart failure will vary, depending on the specific organs that are congested. Generally, swelling—especially in the legs and feet—is common.

*Heart Valve Disease.*

*Congenital Heart Defects.* Defects at birth.

*Tachycardia.* Rapid heartbeat.

## Good Nutrition Helps Control the Risk

For many years, hardening of the arteries was believed to be an irreversible condition, but recent studies have proven otherwise. You *can* reverse the condition if you (1) reduce your cholesterol intake; (2) stop smoking; (3) follow a sensible diet; (4) and change certain habits in your lifestyle.

Generally, a vegetarian diet helps control many of the risk factors associated with heart disease. In studies that compared vegetarians to meat-eaters of similar age and social status, vegetarians showed lower levels of cholesterol, triglycerides, and blood fats. Further, older men who eat meat six or more times a week are four times as likely to have a heart attack and twice as likely to die of heart disease.

But a low-fat diet alone is not the answer. In fact, among certain Africans and Eskimos whose diets are high in animal fats, heart disease is lower than that of most Western populations. Note, however, that in these cultures, people eat no refined or highly processed foods.

To reduce your chances of having cardiovascular disease, follow these recommendations:

• Add plenty of soy products to your diet—soy grits, tofu, tempeh, and soy beans. Soy protein is more effective in lowering blood cholesterol levels than almost any other low-fat, low-cholesterol foods. Also, eat walnuts and seaweed. Like soy, walnuts and seaweed contain omega-3 fatty acids, which may be responsible for lowering blood cholesterol.

• Eat plenty of legumes, including these dried beans: black beans, kidney beans, lentils, chick peas, lima beans, and split peas.

These beans contain a fiber that may block the absorption of certain harmful types of cholesterol.

• Add black tree fungus to your diet. This edible fungus (known as "mo-er"), which commonly is used in Chinese cooking, has anticlotting properties that may account for the low rate of heart attacks in China. Specifically, this fungus contains adenosine, an anticlotting agent also present in garlic and onions. ["Science Watch," *New York Times*, February 17, 1981.]

• Limit your daily sodium intake to one gram for every 1,000 calories, but not more than three grams (about one level teaspoon) a day.

• Avoid all meats.

• Reduce your total cholesterol intake to less than 100 milligrams per 1,000 calories but not more than 300 milligrams a day. When you stop eating meat, do not substitute other high-LDL-containing foods and foods that are high in saturated fats, such as eggs, whole milk, butter, cheese, organ meats, coconut and palm kernel oil, margarine and vegetable shortening, and shrimp. (LDL is explained in greater detail later in the discussion on "Establishing a Risk-Control System" on page 48.)

• Reduce your triglyceride levels by keeping your daily carbohydrate intake between 60 and 90 grams and avoiding all alcoholic beverages and refined sugars.

• Increase your protein intake but avoid high-fat sources of protein. If you include dairy products in your diet, the best choices are yogurt, low-fat or skim milk, and nonfat dried milk. Yogurt may help reduce blood-cholesterol levels.

• Avoid eating hard cheeses. The only low-fat hard cheeses are Swiss, St. Otho, Swiss Sap Sago, German hand cheese, and Norwegian gammelost.

• Include one or two tablespoons of olive oil in your daily diet.

• Snack on raw unsalted seeds, such as sesame, sunflower, and pumpkin.

• Avoid coffee and other caffeinated beverages.

• Increase your intake of raw onions and garlic, both of which can lower high cholesterol levels.

• Increase your fiber intake to at least one ounce a day.

• Be careful of the crackers you eat! Many crackers are high in fat. The American Heart Association lists these fat-free crackers: flat bread, Finn Crisp, hardtack, whole wheat matzos, Swedish crispbread, and Wasa Brod.

• Eat light meals in the evening and heavier meals earlier in the day.

• Increase your intake of fruits, especially apples and berries. Both contain pectin, which reduces the absorption of cholesterol into the bloodstream.

• Eat the following foods liberally:

| | |
|---|---|
| Buckwheat (it's high in rutin) | Potatoes |
| Millet | Okra |
| Raw, unsalted sunflower seeds | Asparagus |
| Hulled sesame seeds | Brewer's yeast |
| Bananas | Flaxseed oil |

## Lifestyle Changes Help Control the Risk

How do you begin to control the risks involved in cardiovascular disease? Follow these recommendations:

*Control Your Blood Pressure.* Follow a diet that will help control your blood pressure. Many experts believe that hypertension is the number one factor in heart disease. When blood pressure remains too high for an extended period, the arteries become damaged, although the damage may not be immediately apparent.

*Stop Smoking.* Cigarette smoking has many detrimental features, some of which were discussed previously.

*Smoking Vs. Nonsmoking.* Smoking reduces the amount of oxygen that your bloodstream carries to your body's cells. Less oxygen forces your heart to work harder in its effort to supply as much oxygen as the body needs. Smoking also narrows your blood vessels and produces gases and chemicals that can cause atherosclerosis. Nicotine reduces the level of prostacyclin, an important chemical that helps protect blood vessels from injury, and thereby increases the chances of damaging the heart. Nicotine also raises your blood pressure and increases your heart rate. If you smoke, make a determined effort to stop!

*Exercise, Exercise, Exercise.* Despite the lack of solid proof that exercise can prevent heart attacks, there is a definite statistical correlation between cardiovascular health and physical activity. Thus exercising is always an essential part of cardiovascular rehabilitation.

*Lose Weight, If Necessary.* People who are overweight by 20 percent or more of their ideal weight are risking heart problems. There are a number of reasons why obesity increases the chances of cardiovascular disease. Simply put, the more weight you carry, the harder your heart must work.

*Control Your Cholesterol Intake.* There are two types of cholesterol: *HDL* ("*high-d*ensity *l*ipoprotein") cholesterol is good for you. Exercise may actually increase your HDL cholesterol levels. *LDL* ("*low-d*ensity *l*ipoprotein") cholesterol is the harmful one.

*Control Stress Factors Around You.* Anger and hostility create stress and contribute to heart disease. Stress conditions force your body to release adrenal hormones, which raise your blood pressure and your heart rate. Thus people under stress will often experience chest pains or heart palpitations. While occasional stress may not cause serious problems, constant stress can be damaging. People who have what is known as a "Type A" personality are especially prone to heart disease. These people react very poorly to stressful situations and have difficulty adapting to their environment.

*Control Your Blood Sugar.* If you are a diabetic, control your blood-sugar levels very carefully, and you will reduce your chances of heart disease. If you do not, you will increase your risk of heart disease.

## Help Your Heart Through Wise Supplementation

A number of supplements are known to be helpful in fighting heart disease:

*Acidophilus.* Acidophilus helps reduce blood cholesterol.

*Activated Charcoal.* A Finnish study shows that taking one-quarter ounce of activated charcoal three times a day for four weeks may lower blood levels of harmful LDL cholesterol.

*Calcium.* At levels of 1,000 milligrams or more daily, calcium can reduce cholesterol levels.

*Carnitine and Magnesium.* Carnitine and magnesium are the two most important nutrients for strengthening the heart. Carnitine can reduce the fatty deposits (triglycerides) that accumulate in and damage arteries. Carnitine can also improve the burning of fats, especially in heart muscle and liver cells, and it may therefore improve the heart muscle's tolerance for exercise.

Magnesium is used to control irregular heartbeats (even after heart attacks). It lowers cholesterol levels and improves the elasticity of blood vessels. A deficiency of magnesium in heart muscle may increase the risk of sudden heart attack.

*Lecithin.* Lecithin keeps cholesterol in solution in the blood, preventing the formation of fatty deposits in the arteries. It reduces levels of harmful LDL and increases levels of beneficial HDL cholesterol. Lecithin is most effective when it is taken as part of a low-fat diet.

*EFAs, Vitamin E, and Pectin.* The essential fatty acids (EFAs)—especially lino-leic acid—and vitamin E also help control blood-cholesterol levels. Vitamin E also improves poor circulation. For years the Shute Institute in Ontario, Canada, has used vitamin E successfully to treat cardiovascular disease. Pectin limits the amount of cho-lesterol that the body absorbs.

*Chromium.* This mineral helps protect against coronary artery disease by reduc-ing cholesterol levels and aortic plaques. Use GTF (*g*lucose *t*olerance *f*actor) chro-mium.

*Vitamin B₆.* Vitamin $B_6$ reduces platelet aggregation and the potential of clot for-mation, a major problem for heart patients.

*Vitamin C.* Vitamin C has many benefits. It (1) reduces plaque levels in the arteries and reduces triglycerides by activating an enzyme called "lipoprotein lipase;" (2) increases the destruction of fibrin, which causes clots, and as a result, makes vita-min C especially helpful for people with a history of heart disease; (3) reduces LDL and increases HDL cholesterol; and (4) helps improve circulation.

*Omega-3 Fatty Acids.* Convincing evidence now points to the beneficial features of omega-3 fatty acids on the heart and cardiovascular system.

## Juice Therapy

For angina, try Juice Therapy Formulas #8 and #19. For arteriosclerosis, try Juice Therapy Formula #20. See Juice Therapy in the Appendix.

## Herbs Are Excellent Remedies

For general heart problems, herbs such as hawthorn berry extract, tincture of cayenne (capsicum), garlic, black cohash, and horsetail (silica tablets) are known to be effec-tive.

Herb remedies may be used effectively for the following specific heart problems:

*Angina.* Among the most popular herbs used to reduce the discomfort of angina are: hawthorn berry, tilia flowers, peruvian bark, siberian ginseng, capsicum, sarsapa-rilla, and lobelia.

*Atrial Fibrillation.* Use cinchona bark, which is the source of quinine.

*Fibrinolytic Activity (FA).* Fibrinolytic activity—"FA" for short—is the process of dissolving small blood clots before they become major blockages in a blood vessel. The body performs this function naturally. Garlic and cayenne pepper (capsicum) help increase FA. Butcher's broom (*Ruscus aculeatus*) is popularly used in Europe to re-duce blood clotting after surgery.

*Heart Palpitations.* Palpitations caused by a nervous response can be reduced by wild cherry bark.

## Aroma Therapy

A number of plant essences are especially useful in aroma therapy:

• For angina pectoris: essence of aniseed, caraway, and orange blossom.

• For arteriosclerosis: essence of garlic, juniper, lemon, and onion.

• For heart spasms: A number of aromatic oils, among them calamus and melissa, have an antispasmodic effect on the heart.

- For heart palpitations: essence of rosemary, aniseed, caraway, orange blossom, and peppermint.
- For tachycardia: essence of ylang-ylang and garlic.

## Exercise Your Heart Muscles

First, check with your physician to make sure that you can exercise safely and that you begin a regular exercise program. With your physician's approval, you can then begin with the least-stressful, most-productive exercises, swimming and walking. Start walking 1 mile; then work your way up to longer distances, say, 3 to 5 miles each day.

## Visualization

Visualization, too, can help relieve angina pains. Use the step-by-step visualization technique described on page 30.

## How Barry R. Fights Angina

Now 50, Barry is well aware that in many ways his former lifestyle was typical of all the successful stockbrokers he knew. He was always under a great deal of stress on the job. He was 20 pounds overweight and too busy to exercise. Barry ate fried foods far too often and usually grabbed lunch on the run. He smoked far too much and drank cup after cup of coffee at his desk. With dinner each evening he had a glass of wine.

Except for an annual cold and occasional headaches, he had never really been ill, that is, not until last year. That's when he started to feel pains around his heart and into his shoulder whenever he ran to the bus in the morning. The first time he felt the pain, he suspected he was having a heart attack and naturally felt rather terrified, enough to make an appointment with a doctor.

The nutritionally oriented physician checked Barry thoroughly and reviewed his personal and family health history in detail, as well as Barry's lifestyle. He discovered that Barry had high blood pressure. The lab reports showed high blood cholesterol and triglyceride levels. The diagnosis was clear: *angina pectoris*.

Barry's physician prescribed no medications but immediately placed him on a general health-building program. The doctor recommended that Barry:

1. Eat a large salad every day.
2. Go on a lacto vegetarian diet, drinking low-fat milk and eliminating all meat, fish, poultry, and eggs.
3. Use whole grains and beans as a source of protein and fiber as well as to reduce blood cholesterol.
4. Walk at least one-half hour a day, three times a week. His doctor had already determined that there was no medical risk to this exercise program.
5. Supplement his diet with vitamins C and E, lecithin, hawthorne berry herbal syrup, omega-3 fatty acids, and plenty of fresh onions and garlic to reduce cholesterol and lower blood pressure.

At first, Barry had difficulty changing his well-formed lifestyle and sticking to his new diet. He occasionally sneaked a greasy fried hamburger or a slice of pizza; but as soon as he realized that he was losing weight, he renewed his commitment to the program. He even gave up his morning coffee and evening wine!

The result? Ten weeks later Barry was "a new man." His heart pains disappeared, he lost 20 pounds, his blood pressure was normal, and his muscles were toned and firm.

In addition to all of his doctor's recommendations, Barry began a stress-management program: he attended massage sessions once a week, he went through 20 minutes of visualization techniques each day, and played racquetball once a week.

Barry still actively fights angina by keeping to his diet and exercise program.

# 10

# Celiac

In the small intestines are *villi*, tiny hairlike objects that project from the intestine wall. Because the villi are responsible for absorbing fluids and nutrients, they perform a very, very important task. When the villi do not perform their job, the body cannot get all the essential nutrients it needs.

Celiac is a condition in which the villi are damaged by gluten, the protein portion of grain. For most people, gluten is a harmless, healthy protein that causes no special problem, but for those afflicted with celiac, the gluten damages the villi for reasons still unknown.

## Celiac Symptoms

The symptoms of celiac disease may include constipation, diarrhea; or stools that are pale, greasy, bulky, or especially odorous. In addition, the following physical disorders may derive as symptoms of celiac disease:

| | |
|---|---|
| Weakness | Iron deficiency anemia |
| Weight loss | Vomiting |
| Poor appetite | Osteomalacia |
| Protruding abdomen | Obesity |
| Scaly skin | Bone pain |
| Cramps and spasms | Very pale skin color |

## Diagnosing Celiac

An accurate diagnosis of celiac disease should be made only by a qualified professional. The process involves examining a minute specimen from the surface of the small intestine. If the specimen shows damage to the villi, then celiac disease is assumed to be the cause, and the treatment should begin immediately. People who suffer from celiac have a high risk of getting cancer of the gastrointestinal tract.

## Foods to Avoid

Understandably, if you suffer from celiac, you must avoid any grains or foods containing gluten including: wheat, barley, malt, rye, and oats.

Be especially careful to avoid foods prepared in Chinese restaurants, where some foods can contain a type of wheat gluten called "seitan." Rice and corn contain no gluten. Some people who suffer from celiac disease cannot handle milk products well.

## Your Supplementation Program

Because celiac specifically prevents the absorption of nutrients, you must be especially sure to supplement your diet. Children who suffer from celiac disease may outgrow the condition as they mature, thus, supplementation is especially important.

Your supplementation program should include:

| | | |
|---|---|---|
| Vitamin A | Vitamin E | Calcium |
| Vitamin B complex | Vitamin C | Magnesium |
| Vitamin D | Folate | Betaine HCL |
| Vitamin K | Iron | Digestive enzymes |
| Vitamin $B_{12}$ | | |

## Also of Interest

Studies show that more children who were breast-fed were able to tolerate gluten. Apparently, the reason lies in the fact that grain is introduced into the diets of breast-fed children much later.

Celiac disease may often be the cause of diarrhea in insulin-dependent diabetics.

# 11

# Dental and Oral Problems

According to Dr. Jerry Mittelmens, there are eight warning signs of gum disease:

1. Bleeding gums when brushing
2. Persistent bad breath
3. Soft, swollen, or tender gums
4. Pus seeping from your teeth when you press on them
5. Loose permanent teeth
6. Receding gums
7. Changes in the way your dentures fit
8. Shifting teeth—that is, change in your bite

[Jerry Mittleman's *Holistic Health Digest*, 263 West End Ave., New York, NY 10023]

Whenever you see such warnings, be sure to take steps to prevent the problem from worsening. Fortunately, many of the most common dental and oral problems can be improved by natural healing.

*Gingivitis.* An invisible bacterial film called *plaque* is constantly forming in your mouth. Plaque that forms along the gumline causes pain, redness, swelling, and irritation. As a result, your gums may bleed when you brush.

If gingivitis is left untreated, the plaque will harden below the gumline and form a rocklike, thorny substance called "tartar." Tartar must be removed by specialized dental instruments, not by simple brushing or flossing.

Gingivitis is an early stage of periodontal disease. Consider it a warning that you must take steps to prevent further damage.

*Pyorrhea.* This is an infectious disease of the tooth sockets and gums. Among the symptoms are loosening of the teeth and the formation of pus.

*Temperomandibular Joint Syndrome (TMJ).* TMJ describes a condition when the joint of the jaw—the temperomandibular joint—and the muscles used for chewing fail to work properly together. As a result, jaw movement may be irregular or limited, you may hear grinding and clicking during movement of the jaw, or you may feel pain and tenderness in the jaw joint. (Many other conditions, such as knee pain, lower-back pain, and headaches, can often be attributed to TMJ.)

What causes TMJ? Stress, poor bite, accidents that have damaged facial or jaw bones, bruxism (described next), or diseases such as arthritis are some causes of TMJ.

*Bruxism* is grinding of the teeth, usually during sleep. As a result of the grinding, the teeth may become loose in their sockets. Bruxism is associated with stress and poor nutrition.

## Good Nutrition Contributes to Dental and Oral Health

Good nutrition works as effectively to keep your teeth and gums healthy as it does for the rest of your body. Here are some general measures for good dental health:

• Eat foods that require plenty of chewing, apples, for example. Apples are excellent for stimulating the gums and cleaning the teeth.

• Avoid foods that are gooey or sticky to chew.

• Be sure that you get enough calcium in your diet. Without calcium, your jawbone can shrink and cause you to lose teeth.

• Eat millet and hulled sesame seeds. They have a high calcium and phosphorus content and are therefore very valuable for dental and oral health.

Now let's see how nutrition can help in specific dental/oral problems:

*For Oral Cavity Inflammation.* Drink the juices of young barley grasses (blue green manna).

*To Prevent Caries (Cavities).* (1) Eat foods that are not cariogenic—that is, that do not cause cavities such as raw vegetables, most fruits, unsalted popcorn, nuts, seeds, and milk products.

(2) Avoid foods that can cause cavities; for example, peaches, pineapples, and oranges because they are high in natural sugar. Also avoid dried fruits such as raisins and apricots. They have a high natural-sugar content and stick to the teeth as well.

(3) Eat at least 1/2 ounce of cheese whenever you do eat foods with a high natural-sugar content. British studies show that cheese can help stop the formation of cavity-causing bacteria in dental plaque.

## Specific Supplements for Specific Problems

Follow these recommendations for specific dental and oral conditions:

*Bruxism.* Take calcium. Because it is effective for treating involuntary muscle movement, calcium may also help bruxism conditions.

*Gum Inflammation.* Vitamin E inhibits certain prostaglandins, which are responsible for gum inflammation.

*Periodontal Disease.* Vitamin C (one gram daily) may help prevent or kill one of the primary bacteria in periodontal disease (actinomyces) and root surface caries, which are common in older people who suffer from receding gums. Propilus is also effective in treating periodontal disease. (See page 25 for more information on propilus.)

*Pyorrhea.* Take vitamin C and bioflavonoids. Rub your gums vigorously with vitamin E. (Break open a capsule of vitamin E, or apply it using a dropper bottle.)

*Dental Caries.* Take molybdenum, which is found primarily in whole grains and some fats. The question of fluoride use is highly controversial. Although fluoridation of water supplies has been shown to reduce caries among young people, most healers favor ingesting fluoride naturally through foods and nutrients rather than artificially through mass medication. There is enough data to support the possibility that fluoridation may promote cancer, kidney disease, birth defects, sickle-cell anemia, heart disease, and immunological deficiencies.

## Juice Therapy

For healthy teeth, drink Juice Therapy Formula #16 (see Appendix) or carrot and other vegetable juices. For pyorrhea, drink one pint of spinach juice daily. Limit your use of fruit juices.

## Use Herbs for Healthy Teeth and Gums

Various herbs are good for oral health. Myrrh and white oak bark are good for dental health. Rubbing lobelia extract onto your gums and rinsing your mouth repeatedly with chamomile tea helps to relieve the pain of toothaches. After a tooth extraction, gargle with chamomile tea.

One toothpaste that supposedly is effective in fighting plaque is Viadent (from Vipont Laboratories in Colorado), which contains a natural plaque-fighting substance extracted from sanguinaria, or blood root plant. "When Viadent toothpaste and mouth rinse were used daily by orthodontic patients, plaque was reduced 53 percent and gum inflammation 50 percent." [Jane E. Brody, "Personal Health," *New York Times*, April 2, 1986.]

Make your own herbal tooth powder as follows: On a stainless steel tray, mix four teaspoons sage leaf, three teaspoons sea salt or rock salt and one teaspoon myrrh. Heat the mixture in an oven at medium temperature for approximately 30 minutes. Remove the tray from the oven and allow the mixture to cool for about 10 minutes. Grind finely to a powder with a mortar and pestle or an electric mill (or use a grain mill or a coffee mill). Press the mixture through a fine sieve; throw out any lumps that remain in the sieve. Store the powder in a dry, dark, cool place. This powder is gently abrasive and has an antibacterial quality.

## Aroma Therapy

Here are two aroma therapy techniques that are useful for dental and oral problems:

- For gingivitis, try oil of lemon and oil and sage.

• For toothaches, apply oil of cloves directly to the painful area. Rinse your mouth with a tea made from cloves.

## How You Can Use Tissue Salts

You can use tissue salts as part of your dental program:

- For general dental health, calcium fluoride 6X is recommended.
- For toothache, calcium phosphate.
- For toothache accompanied by sore gums, calcium fluoride.
- For periodontal disease, potassium phosphate.

## You CAN Prevent Plaque Buildup

To prevent plaque buildup, follow this five-step routine each day:

1. Use special disclosing tablets to stain the plaque on your teeth and make the plaque visible.
2. With a dry, soft-bristle brush, brush daily using a back-and-forth motion. Note that *dry* brushing is recommended—do not use toothpaste. Recent studies show that brushing back and forth is more effective in removing plaque than brushing in an up-and-down-motion. [Jane E. Brody, "Personal Health," *New York Times*, April 2, 1986.]
3. Use unwaxed dental floss to clean under the edge of your gums and between all your teeth.
4. Rinse your mouth. Now look closely at your teeth for any remaining stains.
5. Brush your teeth and tongue again—this time, with toothpaste.

Many dentists consider toothpaste ineffective. Instead, they recommend using baking soda, which reduces halitosis. You may also add a little sea salt to achieve a more-abrasive quality.

## Also of Interest

You may find the following comments helpful in establishing an effective dental program:

- The mercury in silver-mercury amalgam fillings is considered very harmful by a number of doctors and dentists; so much so, that they recommend removing all mercury fillings and replacing them with newer, safer materials.
- If your teeth are stained and yellow, brush with charcoal powder (available in local drugstores). Then place a strawberry on your brush and proceed to brush as usual.

## For More Information

You may wish to contact one or more of the following sources for information on topics of special interest to you:

American Association of Orthodontists
460 North Lindbergh Boulevard
St. Louis, MO 63141

Coalition of Mercury Amalgam Victims
P.O. Box 458
Allston, MA 02134

Toxic Testing, Inc. (1)
303 East Altamonte Drive, Suite 232
Altamonte Springs, FL 32701

American Holistic Dental Association
1-800-231-9834

New York State Coalition Opposed to Fluoridation
P.O. Box 263
Old Bethpage, NY 11804

(1) Toxic Testing compiles a list of dentists who do not use mercury amalgams.

# 12

# Diabetes Mellitus

Diabetes is a chronic disorder that affects the metabolism and involves many of the body's organs. As compared to the normal population, diabetics have a higher potential for circulatory problems, blindness, and gallstones.

In the case of diabetes, the body cannot manufacture an important hormone, insulin, nor can it properly utilize any insulin that it does manufacture. Without insulin, the body's metabolism is upset and imbalanced. First, the body will not be able to metabolize carbohydrates. This malfunction then sets off an intricate chain reaction of other improper bodily functions.

One result is that the level of glucose, a type of sugar, in the blood begins to rise. Eventually, the glucose will be excreted in the urine. Thus one routine test for diabetes is to test the level of sugar in the urine. Once sugar is found in the urine, however, other follow-up tests are essential to diagnose this condition accurately.

## Some Common Symptoms

If you suspect that you have diabetes, you *must* consult your physician. Proper testing is mandatory in diagnosing this condition.

Diabetics may experience many different symptoms, but seldom at the same time. Some common symptoms of diabetes are:

- Excessive thirst
- Frequent urination

- Unexplainable loss of weight
- Bruises, cuts, or infections that take longer than normal to heal
- Constant hunger
- Mood swings
- Excessive fatigue and physical weakness for no apparent reason
- Greater susceptibility to infection (in women, especially vaginal infections)
- A tingling "pins and needles" sensation in the fingers and toes
- Eye problems, including blurred vision and bleeding from the tiny blood vessels in the retina
- Impotence
- Nausea
- Vomiting
- Very dry skin
- Leg cramps
- A sweet breath odor

Although high blood pressure is not a symptom of diabetes, it is often associated with this condition.

## The Two Types of Diabetes

If you are over 40 and overweight, and there is a history of diabetes in your family, your chances of having diabetes are increased. Proper testing will determine which type of diabetes a patient has.

- *Type 1*, also called "juvenile diabetes," is the less-common type. In Type 1 diabetes, the body's special insulin-producing cells (*beta* cells) stop producing insulin. As a result, unless the patient takes insulin injections, Type 1 diabetes can be fatal.
- *Type 2* generally occurs during pregnancy or middle age, especially in over-weight people. In Type 2, the body generally produces some insulin, but its production is inconsistent, and the body is not always able to use this insulin properly. Type 2 diabetics can control their disorder with proper nutrition and good exercise habits.

## Control Your Glucose Levels

The need for careful control of your sugar levels is essential because diabetes can damage the kidneys, nerves, and eyes, and it can cause cardiovascular disease. If you have diabetes and must take insulin, you can control your condition best if you test your own sugar levels regularly.

One test allows you to determine the level of sugar in your urine. A better and more accurate self-test requires you to prick your finger and test a drop of your blood. In both tests, you use a special strip of colored paper to determine your sugar level. Self-testing is especially valuable for pregnant diabetics.

## Nutritional Guidelines for Diabetics

Diabetics must be especially careful to eat sensibly. If you are diabetic, be sure to:

- Eat numerous small meals rather than three large meals each day.

• Prepare meals with more nonstarchy vegetables. Do not rely exclusively on starchy foods like beans, corn, and peas.

• When you do eat starchy vegetables, eat lentils and other beans because they release carbohydrates very slowly.

• Increase your intake of EFAs (essential fatty acids) by adding two tablespoons of sesame, safflower, sunflower, or flaxseed oil to your diet. These EFAs can help your body normalize many of the biochemical abnormalities associated with diabetes.

• Eat high-fiber foods as part of your healing program. High-fiber foods help diabetics to lose weight, and fiber reduces the insulin requirements for some diabetics.

• In many Native American tribes, as well as throughout Latin America, people use de-spined cactus pads as a "cure" for Type 2 diabetes. Hispanic food stores usually carry fresh cactus leaves.

• Eliminate alcohol and tobacco.

## Supplements That Aid Diabetics

A number of supplements are especially valuable for the diabetic.

*DMG.* In studies on diabetic mice, Dr. M. E. Racho of the University of Bridgeport found that the animals who received DMG (dimethylglycine) had lower blood-glucose levels and lower body weight.

*Apple Pectin.* Apple pectin reduces the need for insulin after meals.

*Chromium.* Supplementation with chromium, especially through brewer's yeast, increases healthy glucose control.

*Vitamin C.* Diabetics, especially those who take insulin, lose vitamin C at a higher rate than nondiabetics.

*Vitamin E.* Vitamin E helps increase the healing of gangrene and ulcers.

## Juice Therapy for the Diabetic

If you have diabetes, you will find the following juice therapies very healthy:

• Drink one pint of string bean juice each day.

• Try Juice Therapy Formula #13 (see Appendix).

• Mix and drink the juice of carrots and Jerusalem artichokes (which actually belong to the sunflower family, not the artichoke family). According to N. W. Walker, considered by many to be the pioneer of juice therapy, Jerusalem artichokes contain inulin, a starchlike substance that does not require insulin to be digested by the body.

• Drink cucumber juice. It may contain a plant hormone that helps the pancreas produce insulin.

## Herb Therapy for the Diabetic

The following herbs may have special nutritional value for diabetics:

| | |
|---|---|
| Siberian ginseng | Nettle leaves |
| American ginseng | Skullcap |
| Blueberry leaves | Dandelion |
| Alfalfa | Oregon grape root |
| Horsetail | Licorice root |

| Uva ursi leaves | Goldenseal root |
|---|---|
| Mullein | Garlic |
| Cayenne | Passion flower |

In addition, a Chinese herb, don sen or tang shen (*Campanumaea pilosula*), is used to strengthen the pancreas.

## Massage for the Diabetic

Deep massage may cause nerve or circulatory problems for the diabetic, but gentle massage and gentle kneading are harmless.

## Aroma Therapy

Try using the oils of eucalyptus, geranium, juniper, and onion.

## Exercise for Diabetics

Exercise is of great value for diabetics. For example, doing aerobic exercises regularly can help improve your carbohydrate tolerance. In Type 2 diabetes, exercise increases tissue sensitivity to insulin.

## How Harold H. Fought Off Gangrene

Harold H., now 75 years old, came dangerously close to having his leg amputated and losing his eyesight. It was just four years ago that Harold began taking his Type 2 diabetes seriously. Until then, his general health habits were very poor.

One day he noticed a blood-filled boil on his toe, but he ignored the boil. The boil then turned black. Only when his family prodded him, did Harold finally visit his family physician, who immediately diagnosed the condition as gangrene and hospitalized Harold. Hospital tests showed Harold's blood-sugar level was dangerously high. Even with insulin, his blood-sugar level was hard to control. His gangrene spread through the toes on his left foot, and the toes had to be surgically removed. When the gangrene spread to the foot itself, the doctors discussed the possibility of amputating his leg at the knee.

Instead, Harold was transferred to another hospital to try a new experimental approach, *hyperbaric oxygen therapy*. The treatment involved placing Harold in a special room where oxygen was introduced at high pressures. At the same time, Harold began a nutritional program that included string beans, blueberry leaf tea, vitamin E (for circulation), tissue salts, Jerusalem artichoke juice, and GTF chromium (to increase pancreatic function).

Along with this new therapy and his new nutritional program, Harold received insulin injections and used visualization techniques to help heal his left leg. Specifically, he would visualize the high-pressure oxygen going into the gangrenous tissue and turning the flesh from black and green to a healthy pink color.

Together, the treatment, the nutritional program, the visualization techniques, and the insulin contributed to Harold's progress in controlling his condition. Within three weeks, the doctors and surgeons were amazed. Harold's gangrenous tissue began to heal, his blood-sugar level dropped, and the circulation in his legs improved.

# 13

# Digestive Disorders

More than any other health problems, digestive disorders respond very well to natural healing methods. The digestive tract is a 30-foot-long tube that digests food and absorbs nutrients. Digestion begins in the mouth, where chewing breaks food into smaller pieces while the saliva begins to break down complex carbohydrates and starches into sugars, and ends with the elimination of waste materials.

Different parts of this long tube perform different functions, and branching off from the tube are various organs and glands that contribute to the digestive process; for example, the pancreas, the liver, and the gallbladder. When any of the many mechanical or chemical processes involved in digestion break down, we experience one or more of the many different symptoms that warn us about a digestive disorder.

## Symptoms of Digestive Disorders

Also known as gastrointestinal disorders, digestive problems generally become noticeable as a result of symptoms such as cramping, burning, growling, pain, churning, and bloating.

When such symptoms become worse or return frequently, then you should consult a competent health professional. You should also consult a professional if you:

- Have difficulty swallowing food.
- Feel pain when swallowing.
- Find blood in your vomit.
- Find mucus or pus in your stools.

- Have unexplainable, recurring pain lasting six hours or more accompanied by fever, chills, shaking, and cold, clammy skin.
- Experience bowel movement changes—for example, a sudden change from diarrhea to constipation, extreme color changes in the stool, and so on.
- Notice a yellow coloring of the skin and eyes than cannot be associated with normal beta carotene supplementation (not more than 75,000 iu daily) or with an intake of carrot juice. The yellow coloring might indicate jaundice.
- See dark, tea-colored urine that cannot be associated with a high intake of B vitamins.
- Have an unexplainable fever over 101 degrees Fahrenheit for two days or more.

## Common Causes

The most common causes of digestive disorders are:

- Overeating.
- Eating too rapidly and not chewing your food sufficiently.
- Nutritional deficiencies, especially those resulting from ingesting large amounts of refined carbohydrates and other processed foods.
- Using coffee, tea, alcohol, and tobacco products.
- Low levels of hydrochloric acid (possibly the result of a niacin deficiency).
- Eating very spicy foods.

## How Good Nutrition Can Help Ease Digestive Problems

Proper nutrition can be exceptionally helpful in both preventing and treating digestive disorders.

*Fast.* Fasting is very helpful in all digestive conditions except stomach ulcers.

*Avoid Spicy Foods.* When you are suffering from a digestive disorder, avoid spicy foods, coffee, green and black teas, and alcohol. In acute conditions, avoid high-fiber foods.

*Try Cultured Foods.* Cultured foods prevent intestinal putrefaction and are very effective healers for people suffering from virtually any digestive problems. Cultured foods include sauerkraut, kefir, sourdough bread, yogurt, and buttermilk.

*Add Fiber.* Many gastrointestinal disorders can be traced to the patient's diet; specifically, to diets high in refined foods and low in essential fiber. Vegetarians are less likely to suffer from gastrointestinal diseases, especially diverticular disease, probably because their diets are rich in cereal fiber.

A low-fiber diet is best while the condition is inflamed, but after this acute stage, a high-fiber diet is best. Raw millers bran, whole grains, and beans are good sources of dietary fiber, but they should be taken in moderation and with plenty of fluids. To avoid complications, be sure to limit your use of bran to 2 to 5 tablespoons daily.

*Drink Distilled Water.* If you have digestive problems, drink distilled water. Any of the many different chemicals in tap water might aggravate—or possibly cause—a digestive problem.

*Eat Salads.* At the end of a meal, especially after eating proteins, be sure to eat salads. The salad will enable the protein-digesting acids and enzymes to function without interference from carbohydrates, which are digested by other enzymes.

*Food Combining.* Avoid mixing fruits and vegetables at the same meal. Limit the combination of carbohydrates and proteins at the same meal.

Now let's see how nutrition can help in specific digestive disorders:

*Abdominal Gas.* To reduce abdominal gas, follow these suggestions:

1. Eliminate raw fruits and vegetables for a while. Instead, drink fresh vegetable juices and lower-fiber foods such as peeled fruits, bananas, and avocados.

2. Avoid foods that are known to cause gas—bananas, milk, cucumbers, beans, peas, and vegetables in the cabbage family (broccoli, cauliflower, and brussels sprouts).

3. Use activated charcoal capsules. When used in moderation, charcoal is very effective in eliminating gas, but excessive use can deplete essential minerals from your system.

*Colitis.* With this condition, a high-fiber diet is not necessarily recommended, especially if the source of fiber is whole grain. The reason is that in colitis cases, the roughage is poorly digested and can cause fermentation in the bowels, resulting in gas and bowel irritation.

Eat small meals several times a day, rather than a few large meals. Eat yogurt and millet, and experiment by including bananas in your diet on a regular basis. You may want to try a juice fast for a week or so, especially in the case of mucous colitis.

*Diarrhea.* If you suffer from diarrhea, raw carrots can be very helpful.

*Diverticular Disease.* To avoid diverticular disease, avoid constipation. Eat high-fiber foods: millet, brown rice, buckwheat, oats, and foods rich in lactic acid.

*Heartburn.* To fight off the effects of heartburn, eat unprocessed raw millers bran. Also, be sure to avoid alcohol, chocolate, coffee (both decaffeinated and regular coffee), tobacco products, citrus fruits, fried foods, spicy foods, tomatoes, and foods containing tomatoes.

The nicotine in tobacco products aggravates heartburn by forcing sphincter pressure to drop, allowing a brining up of stomach acid.

*Hiatal Hernia.* Avoid all products containing caffeine. Also avoid alcohol, spicy foods, and high-fat foods.

*Lactose Intolerance.* Avoid milk and milk products—except those foods that have reduced lactose levels, such as buttermilk, yogurt, cottage cheese, and kefir (a liquid yogurt-like beverage). In fact, you should even limit the amount of lactose—reduced foods that you consume.

You can take special tablets whenever you do consume lactose-rich foods. For information on obtaining these tablets, see "For More Information" at the end of this section.

*Ulcers.* If you have ulcers, there are a number of general recommendations you should heed whenever the condition is active.

Avoid high-fiber foods, including raw fruits and vegetables, whole grains, breads, nuts, seeds, and cereals. In addition, avoid coffee, alcohol, tobacco products, and milk. Although milk may initially coat the stomach lining, it will also decrease stomach acid and aggravate the situation.

Do not fast during an active or acute phase of ulcers.

You will probably tolerate these foods well: avocados, yams, bananas, white potatoes, and squash.

Also, you might try this mixture: Blend a handful of blanched almonds with a little barley malt syrup and distilled water. Pour the blend through a strainer. Drink the remaining liquid.

For duodenal ulcers olive oil—1 tablespoon 3 times a day for as long as one year—has been helpful.

Certain types of fiber both (1) prevent the formation of ulcers and, at the same time, (2) prevent relapses effectively. The foods that best provide this type of fiber are millet, raw millers bran, and beans.

Remember that these foods should *not* be eaten during the active phase of duodenal ulcers.

If you have ulcerative colitis, food allergies may be contributing to your condition. Avoid milk products, wheat, corn, oats, barley, and rye.

## Supplement Your Diet

The supplements that are most beneficial for specific gastrointestinal conditions are:

*For Colitis:* Vitamins A and C, folate, zinc, and pantothenic acid. These healing nutrients are, interestingly, the same nutrients that are found to be deficient in colitis sufferers!

*For Flatulence:* Pantothenic acid.

*For Gastroduodenal Ulcers:* (stress ulcers in burn patients) Injections of 10,000 to 400,000 iu of water-soluble vitamin A daily has been effective for burn patients, according to Dr. Merill S. Chernov, who presented his findings at the Fourth Annual Meeting of the American Burn Association.

*For Heartburn:* A combination of sodium alginate and calcium/magnesium tablets.

*For Peptic Ulcers:* Follow the nutritional recommendations in the section on "Hypoglycemia," page 105. Many people who suffer from peptic ulcers also have hypoglycemia.

*For Ulcers:* Follow these recommendations:

1. Avoid all foods that stimulate the flow of digestive acids in the stomach: coffee, alcohol, and spicy foods.

2. Do not take aspirin, Alka Seltzer, the ascorbic-acid form of vitamin C, milk, and antacids that contain calcium carbonate. All these substances increase the flow of acid and may aggravate the condition.

3. Take vitamins A and E together. They may help protect against ulcers caused by stress.

4. For gastric ulcers, use green magma, the dried juice of young barley plants.

5. Supplement with zinc.

## Amino Acid Therapy

If you have peptic ulcers, you will find glutamine helpful. It has an antacid quality.

## Juice Therapy for Digestive Problems

For all gastrointestinal disorders, you may take Juice Therapy Formulas #1 and #4 (see the Appendix). In addition, you may drink fresh papaya, wheatgrass, pineapple, or lemon juice. If you wish, you can mix whey with your juices, or you can buy Biota brand juices, which already contain whey.

Here are some juice remedies for specific conditions:

*For Amoebic Dysentery:* Garlic juice.

*For Colitis:* Papaya juice and raw cabbage juice. Also, follow the juice program for ulcers, listed next. Avoid citrus juices.

*For Ulcers:* Combine 12 ounces of carrot juice with 4 ounces of cabbage juice and drink the mixture once a day for one week. After one week, slowly increase the amount of cabbage juice in the mixture from 4 to 12 ounces.

Also mix raw potato and cabbage juice and drink the combination immediately after extraction; otherwise, the mixture loses the healing value of vitamin U.

*For Constipation and Ulcers:* Five times a day, drink 3 ounces of celery juice mixed with 3 ounces of cabbage juice. Also, each day drink 1 pint of spinach juice, the most powerful juice for relieving constipation.

*For Sluggish and Prolapsed Colon:* Drink sorrel juice, which is available at Jamaican food stores.

## Use Herbs for Relief

The herbs that are used for general digestive complaints are chamomile, peppermint, flaxseed, slippery elm, and aloe vera gel.

Herbs that are used for specific problems are:

*For Heartburn:* Ginger, caraway seed, fennel, sage, fresh celery stalks, chamomile, dandelion, and yarrow.

*For Abdominal Pains and Colic in Children:* Catnip, fennel seed, peppermint, lobelia, anise, and ginger. Also for colic, each day try a mixture of 3 cups of chamomile and fennel (mixed half and half).

*For Colitis:* Slippery elm gruel.

*For Dyspepsia:* Gentian, chamomile flowers, angelica root, and lemon balm.

*For Nausea:* Comfrey, oat straw, slippery elm bark, and ginger. Also try 2 cups a day of this mixture: raspberry leaf, ginger root, peppermint leaf, and lemon balm. Another remedy is to chew a clove slowly.

*For Ulcers:* Slippery elm gruel. Also, drink comfrey tea on an empty stomach.

NOTE: Overuse of spicy herbs, may tax your digestive system! Most digestive herbs increase the flow of digestive juices.

## Aroma Therapy

The process of digestion begins when we smell the foods we are about to eat. The aroma stimulates our digestive juices. The better foods smell, the more enjoyable they will taste and the more digestible they will be!

Herbs and spices not only help make foods taste better; they also make them smell better. Here are some aroma therapy suggestions for specific digestive disorders:

*For Colic:* Essence of aniseed (infantile), bergamot, hyssop, and peppermint.

*For Flatulence:* Essence of aniseed, caraway, clove, peppermint, ginger, fennel, coriander, hyssop, peppermint.

*For Intestinal Cramps in Children:* Essence of chamomile.

*For Colitis and Gastroenteritis:* Essence of basil, bergamot, cajeput, chamomile, cinnamon, garlic, geranium, hyssop, lavender, lemongrass, niaoli, rosemary, terebinth, thyme, and ylang-ylang.

*For Constipation:* Essence of cinnamon, fennel, marjoram, and rosemary. Bornea camphor strengthens peristalsis.

*For Acid Indigestion:* Essence of clove, black pepper, and cinnamon leaf contain engenol, which counteracts excess acidity by raising the pH of gastric juices.

*For Parasites in the Intestines:* Essence of bergamot, cajeput, chamomile, caraway, cinnamon, clove, eucalyptus, fennel, garlic, hyssop, lavender, lemon, niaoli, onion, peppermint, savory, rosemary, terebinth, thyme and ylang-ylang.

*For Ulcers* (both gastric and intestinal): Essence of chamomile, geranium, and lemon.

## Acupressure and Massage

Try acupressure and massage for digestive disorders. See the Appendix entitled Homeopathy for more information concerning acupressure and digestive disorders.

- For general disorders, try kneading the abdomen. Also, massage along the dorsal and lumbar spine with aromatic oils.
- To treat gastric ulcers, apply deep rhythmic pressure to both wrists.

## Hydrotherapy

Try these hydrotherapy techniques:

*For Abdominal Gas:* Apply a hot water bottle to your abdomen. Apply a cold shower spray to the abdomen.

*For Vomiting and Diarrhea:* Place on the abdomen compresses made half and half with apple cider vinegar and water.

*For General Stomach Upset:* Place warm compresses over the stomach and abdominal area.

## Understand and Control Emotional Factors

Depression or fear can slow down your digestive activity. On the other hand, anger can increase the secretion of acid into the stomach, and this excess acid can break down the stomach wall and cause ulcers.

Learn and use the techniques discussed in this book to control your emotions!

## Homeopathy

Try these homeopathy remedies:

For General Digestive Problems: Arsenicum.

For Indigestion: Bryonia.

For Abdominal Gas: Chamomilia.

For Vomiting Blood: Arsenicum.

For Vomiting Caused by Overeating: Antimonium crudum.

## Tissue Salts

The tissue salts that are most helpful in digestive disorders are:

*For Colic:* Magnesium phosphate 6X with warm water every 10 minutes until the pain subsides.

*For Improving Poor Digestion:* Calcium phosphate 6X and potassium phosphate 6X.

*After Eating Rich, Fatty Foods:* Alternate taking potassium chloride and phosphate of iron.

*For Heartburn and Yellow-Coated Tongue:* Sodium phosphate. If this does not work, then take these remedies together: magnesium phosphate, sodium phosphate, sodium sulphate, and silicic oxide.

*For Flatulence and Colic:* Magnesium phosphate with hot fennel or ginger tea. If this does not work, then take these remedies together: calcium phosphate, magnesium phosphate, sodium phosphate, and sodium sulfate.

*For Nausea and Vomiting:* Sodium sulfate 6X or phosphate of iron.

## Also of Interest

The following suggestions and recommendations are related to good digestive health:

*For Proper Digestion.* Always allow at least two to three hours of rest from the time you finish dinner to the time you go to bed. Do not wear tight clothing either during or directly after meals. Apply the visualization exercises on page 30.

*For Constipation.* To relieve constipation, exercise regularly, eat plenty of high-fiber foods, and drink fluids regularly throughout the day.

*To Offset the Imbalance Caused by Antibiotics.* Use acidophilus to enhance natural immunity, improve digestion, and increase nutrient absorption, especially of the B vitamins. Acidophilus is very helpful in gastrointestinal conditions caused by antibiotics. Antibiotics upset the helpful bacteria that are naturally found in the bowels. Acidophilus helps to correct the imbalance caused by antibiotics.

*For Diarrhea in Infants.* Carob powder has been found to be effective for diarrhea in infants.

*For Heartburn.* Avoid taking antacids, which usually contain aluminum compounds. Long-term use of antacids with aluminum compounds may deplete your body's calcium and cause bone injury and pain. Also, eat small meals, and avoid lying down after meals.

*For Vomiting in Infants.* To stop habitual vomiting in infants, add carob powder to their milk formulas.

*For Intestinal Gas.* Take about ½ teaspoon of raw Irish potato, chew it well, then swallow it. You will find that this remedy relieves abdominal gas. NOTE: Do *not* try this remedy if you have osteoarthritis.

*For Colitis.* For relief of your colitis pain, add catalyst-altered water to your drinking water, or just take 1 teaspoon of catalyst-altered water each day.

## How False Advertising Hurt Leslie K.

Leslie K. works as an office manager for a newspaper. Now 40, he has a very hectic job—lots of pressure, daily deadlines, and constant movement.

Leslie knows quite a bit about nutrition and tries to eat well. Nonetheless, despite his generally good nutritional habits, he suffered often from diarrhea, heartburn, and bloating. One day, he decided to follow a strict program of high-fiber foods and supplements, but his condition did not improve.

When Leslie read an article about lactose intolerance and milk allergy, he thought he had found the solution. He cut out milk and all milk products and substituted "nondairy" soy cheeses for the cheeses he usually ate. He used nondairy coffee creamer in his herb tea.

Shortly, his condition improved, but it did not clear up completely. Leslie even began exercising and meditating to reduce stress, but still his condition did not clear up altogether. He still felt abdominal and digestive discomfort. What else could he do? Leslie resigned himself to the fact that his condition could not be cured.

Then one day Leslie read an article in a magazine that explained clearly why he had only so-so results. He learned from the article that even certain products labeled "nondairy" and "milk-free" may actually contain some milk! The article specifically mentioned soy cheeses and nondairy coffee creamers.

That was it!

Leslie learned which products were *really* "nondairy" and "milk-free" and used them exclusively. Once he stopped using the phony, mislabeled products, his remaining symptoms disappeared.

## For More Information

To find out more about ways to improve your digestive health, you may find the following sources helpful:

Lactaid Inc. (1)
Pleasantville, NJ 08232

Malabar Formulas
28537 Neuvo Valley Drive
P.O. Box 3
Nuevo, CA 92367

Milk Gest
Gides-Nulife Inc.
Orange, CA 92667

Schiff Bio-Food Products (2)
Moonachie, NJ 07074

(1) For information about Lactaid and other products that will help if you cannot digest lactose.
(2) Makers of Lactozyme powder.

# 14

# Ear Disorders

Many people who suffer from ear disorders find that their conditions improve when they adopt sensible nutritional habits.

## Common Disorders

Before we list some specific techniques for promoting ear health through nutrition, let's review the ear problems that most commonly afflict people.

*Earwax Buildup.* Earwax is a slightly acidic, fatty lubricant secreted by specialized glands. Earwax production is natural, and earwax itself is beneficial; it prevents bacteria from growing in the ear cavity. But when the wax builds up in the ear, it may solidify somewhat and cause hearing problems and discomfort.

*Earache.* Common earaches may be caused by boils, fevers, or a wax buildup.

*Ménière's Disease.* This disorder affects the inner ear. The symptoms of Ménière's disease are hearing ringing sounds, vertigo, nausea, vomiting, and recurring attacks of hearing loss.

*Tinnitus.* Tinnitus can be caused by heavy aspirin use, quinine (even the amount in tonic water, if you drink tonic water excessively), exposure to loud noise, an accumulation of earwax, hypertension, blows to the head, allergies, inner-ear diseases, certain prescription drugs, or hypoglycemia.

Some healers believe that tobacco, caffeine, alcohol, and hallucinogenic drugs contribute to tinnitus, but insufficient research has been conducted so far.

## Good Nutrition Helps Ear Problems

The value of good nutrition in promoting ear health is clear:

- Eat low-fat foods to reduce earwax. Avoid eating high-fat foods such as coconut, avocado, butter, and fried foods. Begin a modified raw food diet using only low-fat products. (See page 23 for information on a modified raw food diet.)

• Eliminate refined sugars and starches, concentrated sweets, and highly processed packaged food products.

## Add Supplements to Your Diet

Specific supplements can help you in these three cases:

*For Earwax Buildup (Ceruminosis):* Supplement with EFAs. Wax may build up because of a deficiency in EFAs.

*For Ear Infection:* Take vitamins A and C.

*For Ménière's Disease:* Take vitamin B complex, vitamins $B_1$ and $B_2$, bioflavonoids, and niacin (100 to 250 milligrams daily for up to 14 days). NOTE: Do not be frightened if you happen to experience a "niacin flush," which is itching, redness and the feeling of having a sunburn. This usually passes in an hour.

Include the following in developing your daily supplementation program: vitamin A, vitamin C, calcium, EFAs, vitamin E, vitamin D, and magnesium.

## Use Herbs for Earaches and Earwax Buildup

For general ear problems, use echinacea or valerian. For earaches or earwax buildup, put one or two drops of mullein, flower oil, or warm castor oil in the affected ear; then place cotton in the ear.

## Aroma Therapy for Ear Problems

For earaches, use oil of cajeput or oil of garlic. For ear inflammations, use oil of lemon or oil of niaouli.

## Hydrotherapy for Earaches

Follow any of these hydrotherapy remedies for earaches:

• Place an onion poultice on your neck. Apply the poultice to the ear to relieve pain and control any discharge from the ear.

• Syringe the ear with warm infusions of chamomile tea, marigold tea, or lemon balm.

• The Meskwaki Indians crushed and simmered ginger root to create an ear poultice. The Winnebago Indians poured into the ear the warm tea that results from steeping the entire yarrow plant. [Dian Dincin Buchman, *Herbal Medicine: The Natural Way to Get Well and Stay Well*, Gramercy Publishing Co., N.Y. 1979, pp. 147–148.]

## Homeopathy

Here are some helpful homeopathy remedies you might try:

*For General Earaches:* Use aconite for a sudden earache that results after a chill or exposure to the cold. If warm compresses make the pain feel worse and you feel irritable, use chamomilia.

*For Inflammations of the Middle Ear:* Use pulsatilla, belladonna, sulfur, or *Mercurius solubilis.*

*For Septic Infections:* Use lachesis 12X

*For Ear Discharges:* Use alternately silicea 12X and causticum.

## Tissue Salts That Bring Relief

When you have an earache, try using the following tissue salts for relief:

- If you have pain and the ear is inflamed, use ferrous phosphate, magnesium phosphate, or silicea.
- If you have pain and swelling, use potassium chloride.
- If you have ear pain and a discharge is present, use calcium sulphate.

## Also of Interest

Note the following comments:

*Earwax Buildup.* Avoid using cotton swabs: they really do not remove earwax; moreover; they can damage the ear. Also avoid using most of the commercial products that claim to clear out earwax; many merely cause the wax to swell. If you wish, use one of the glycerol preparations to soften earwax. Better yet, your physician can easily remove accumulated earwax with a very simple procedure.

*Smoking and Hearing Loss.* Apparently, there is a direct correlation between smoking and hearing loss, perhaps because smoking causes atherosclerosis, which reduces blood flow to the ear. Furthermore, a study at the University of Washington School of Medicine shows that children who are exposed to tobacco smoke at home on a daily basis are more likely to develop persistent fluid in the middle ear.

# 15

# Emotional Health

Perhaps as many as 90 percent of all physical problems have psychological roots at their source.

"Clinical observations . . . suggest that the onset and progress of many diseases—diabetes, multiple sclerosis, myasthenia gravis and cancer among them—are influenced by the psychological state of the patient." [Malcolm W. Browne, "Taking Stock of Cancer Risks: The List Goes On," *New York Times*, February 4, 1985, Section C, p. 5]

But just as physical disorders can result from emotional problems, the reverse, too, is possible: emotional problems can result from physical disorders. For example, anxiety, depression, and emotional fatigue often result from physical conditions. Often, because an emotional condition has no obvious cause, the "diagnosis" may be that the condition is purely emotional while the real reason may be allergies, lighting, ion levels, and so on.

Let's take a closer look at some of today's most common emotional problems, beginning with anxiety disorders.

## What Are "Anxiety Disorders"?

Many people suffer a marked fear or a persistent anxiety concerning a place, an event, a situation, another person, or just about anything else. For example, a man may have a fear of going alone into public places, or a woman may have panic attacks. Most of the

74

time, the reasons why people have such feelings are often not at all clear. There seems to be no real reason why each person should feel any anxiety.

But the symptoms of such disorders are real. The person who suffers from anxiety disorder might feel chest pains, a smothering sensation, dizziness, a feeling of faintness, sweating, hot and cold flashes, blurred vision, or a tingling in the arms and legs.

As you can see, these symptoms imitate quite closely some of the symptoms of heart attacks. But *why* do these people feel anxiety?

We do know that anxiety can be caused by:

*Caffeinism.* An excessive intake of coffee, chocolate, certain teas, and colas can cause caffeinism, which affects people differently, according to each individual's personality. Introverted people are hindered by caffeine in the morning, because the caffeine overstimulates them and interferes with their ability to reason. Impulsive, extroverted people respond better to caffeine because they need more time to wake up mentally in the morning.

*Cerebral Allergies.* These are allergies caused by foods such as milk, peanuts, wheat, and certain food additives.

*Hypoglycemia.* See "Hypoglycemia," which begins on page 105.

*Hyperlipidemic Dementia.* This is a mental disorder associated with high levels of fat in the blood.

But there are surely other causes that we now know little or nothing about. For example, genetic predisposition and heavy-metal poisoning may cause anxiety in some cases.

## How Can Anxiety Be Treated?

The results from treating anxiety through nutritional, behavioral,and psychotherapeutic means are mixed, at best. But as Dr. John C. Pecknold said at the annual meeting of the Canadian Psychiatric Association, "behavior therapy is as effective as benzodiazepines for general anxiety disorders." [*Family Practice News,* February 15–29, 1984.] Some of the more successful therapies are as follows.

*Psychotherapy.* In psychotherapy, the therapist's goal is twofold: (1) to help the patient understand the underlying cause of his or her anxiety and then (2) to overcome the anxiety. Psychotherapy can be effective in treating chronic, moderate anxiety conditions and simple phobias.

*Behavior Therapy.* Instead of addressing the cause of the condition directly, behavior therapy attempts to modify the patient's behavior relating to that condition. For example, if someone is afraid of snakes, behavior therapy tries to relax the patient and at the same time bring the person in close contact with a snake. Studies show that behavior therapy can be successful up to 75 percent of the time in patients who suffer from a simple and clearly defined phobia. Biofeedback can be a valuable tool in applying this approach.

*Art, Music, and Dance Therapy.* These therapies use the creative process to try to reinforce an individual's self-esteem and establish a positive identity. Moreover, these healing approaches clearly do *not* label someone as "mentally ill." Singing, listening to, playing and discussing music are all safe and appropriate means for emotionally disturbed people to communicate with others.

*Pet Therapy.* The responsibility of caring for a pet and the unconditional love that animals, particularly dogs, offer their masters are powerful healing tools. Pet therapy is especially helpful for people who feel isolated and lonely, out of touch with their emotions, and unloved.

*Orthomolecular Psychiatry.* Dr. Linus Pauling coined the term *orthomolecular psychiatry* and describes it as follows:

> The treatment of mental disease by the provision of the optimum molecular environment of the mind, especially the optimum concentrations of substances normally present in the human body.*

Often described as *megavitamin therapy*, orthomolecular psychiatry is based on research studies showing that vitamins, minerals, and biochemical imbalances may be involved in various emotional disorders. For example, in one famous 1952 study, Drs. Abraham Hoffer and Humphrey Osmond achieved many positive results in treating schizophrenia and other mental and emotional disorders with very high dosages of vitamin C, niacin, and other vitamins.

Over the years this approach has been expanded to the treatment of alcoholism, depression, and heart problems.

*Dietary Therapy.* People who suffer from hypoglycemia and wheat allergies or experience reactions to certain food additives, may not be able to fill specific nutritional requirements through normal food sources and normal diets. These disorders have been implicated in various emotional problems, particularly in anxiety disorders. Thus dietary therapy offers an alternative approach to traditional treatments of anxiety disorders and other mental health problems.

## Using Nutrition to Combat Mental and Emotional Problems

You *can* use nutrition to help overcome various mental health problems:

*Agoraphobia.* Take vitamin B complex, vitamins C and E, and lecithin. Have yourself tested for hypoglycemia and allergies.

*Depression.* Depression may have different causes:

1. *Hypoglycemia.* Get yourself tested for hypoglycemia. If you have hypoglycemia, increase your consumption of whole grain and brans. Eat small meals (as many as 6 a day). Avoid refined sugar and white flour products. Reduce your overall caloric intake.

2. *Low digestive acids.* When digestive acids are low, your body will have difficulty assimilating nutrients. Take one teaspoon of apple cider vinegar and water before each meal.

3. *Vitamin $B_{12}$ deficiency.* Supplement with 50 mcg of vitamin $B_{12}$.

4. *Epilepsy.* You don't have to have seizures to have epilepsy. Instead of seizures, some epileptics may experience behavioral abnormalities.

*Schizophrenia.* Eliminate all foods containing gluten. Because certain groups of schizophrenics have a higher rate of celiac disease, the gluten-free program described in "Foods to Avoid" on page 53 is highly recommended.

---

* Carl C. Pfieffer, Ph.D, M.D. *Mental and Elemental Nutrients.* 1975, Keats Publishing, New Canaan, Conn.

## Use Your Human Potential!

The way you view your life will very strongly influence your health. If you have a poor attitude in every situation, your health will suffer from your attitude. If you believe that life is beautiful and that life is to be fully enjoyed, despite occasional upsets, then your health will reflect that attitude.

Remember, your human potential is unlimited. You *can* control the way you view your life! In order to heal, you must have a healing attitude. What is a "healing attitude"? A healing attitude is the ability to see all things as possible even if you do not understand specifically *how* they are possible. In other words, you must view yourself as a healing organism.

Admittedly, a healing attitude takes time to develop. To begin, you should:

1. Get involved in small-group activities and service organizations. By supporting other people, you help them to heal. At the same time, you benefit by learning about the need for support in the healing process!

2. Become involved with friends and family. Ask them for support when you need it, and let them know that you're ready to provide them with support when they need it.

3. Make conscious decisions in choosing your work environment and your play environment.

4. Expand your interests; try new things; learn about new ideas; make new friends and acquaintances. Studies show that having a variety of interests can increase your life span.

5. Bring humor into your life. Spend time with people who love to laugh and help you to laugh. Read humorous books and listen to humorous records and tapes.

6. Look around you for things that you are grateful for. When something unpleasant happens, consider the situation as a test. Apply your skills to change the situation. If it cannot be changed, learn how to adjust to the new situation.

7. Express your feelings freely whenever possible. Holding your feelings in may contribute to feelings of hopelessness and powerlessness. Various illnesses, including cancer, have been associated statistically with individuals who have held back anger all their lives.

## Supplements That Will Help Depression

To help relieve depression, consider the following supplements:

• Vitamin $B_{12}$ injections (administered by a physician) and digestive aids to increase the absorption of nutrients help in treating depression. Also, whenever you take vitamin $B_{12}$, always take folic acid as well.

• Many other B vitamins and vitamin C produce a positive response in certain types of depression. Take vitamin $B_6$, niacinamide, and folate.

## Amino Acid Therapy

Amino acids, too, are helpful in treating various emotional and mental disorders.

*For Depression:* Tyrosine (controls medication-resistant depression), GABA (gama-aminobutyric acid), D-Phenylalanine (both alone and in combination with tyrosine), vitamin $B_6$ and L-Tryptophan (for premenstrual depression).

*For Obsessive and Compulsive Behavior:* L-Tryptophan
*For Insomnia and Depression:* L-Tryptophan
*For Manic Behavior and Acute Agitation:* GABA
*For Schizophrenia:* Tryptophan and Arginine (CAUTION: Arginine should be used only under a physician's guidance.)

## Helpful Herbs

Herbs that you might consider are buchu, hops, pleurisy root, and valerian.

NOTE: Valerian should be used with caution by anyone prone to manic depression.

## Aroma Therapy

According to Dr. Gary Schwartz, professor of psychology and psychiatry at Yale, "Any disorder for which relaxation techniques have been shown to have effectiveness may also respond to aroma therapy." [*New York Times*, January 27, 1985, Section F, p. 17.]

Essences which long have been used to treat depression include basil, peppermint oil, bergamot, geranium, Borneo camphor, chamomile, lavender, and thyme.

## Homeopathy

Try the following homeopathy remedies:
*For Nervousness and Stress:* Arnica
*For Changeable Moods:* Ignatia
*For Nervousness and Anxiousness:* Silicea
*For General Emotional Stress and Fear:* Rescue remedy, also known as Bach remedy (available in concentrated form in most health food stores and better pharmacies)

See the Appendix for a complete list of the Bach Flower Remedies, which are helpful for many different ailments.

## Also of Interest

The following comments on various emotional disorders may also be helpful:
*Tissue Salts.* Phosphate of iron, a tissue salt, is helpful for nervousness.
*Anger and Heart Attacks.* Anger has been clearly associated with heart attacks. For example, in a 25-year study, men with hostile personalities were found to have a risk of heart attack five times greater than nonhostile men. Hostility may be a key part of the Type A personality, which researchers have identified as more likely to suffer from heart disease. If you want to live longer and healthier, learn to control your anger.
*Phobias and the Inner Ear.* According to Dr. Harold Levinson, there may be a connection between inner-ear problems and various space-related phobias, such as fear of flying on airplanes, riding in buses, driving cars, and playing sports. "When the inner ear is unstable," he says, "Patients project their own disoriented gyroscope onto the environment around them. . . ." [*Insight*, September 1, 1986.]

## For Your Information

You may find some of the following resources helpful for information on emotional disorders:

Academy of Orthomolecular Psychiatry
North Nassau Mental Health Center
1691 Northern Boulevard
Manhasset, New York 11030

Make Choices, Not Excuses
The Harrison Institute
40 West 72 Street
New York, NY 10023

Brain Bio Center
1225 State Road
Princeton, NJ 08540
(609) 924-6033

Earth House Inc. (1)
P.O. Box 202
East Millstone, NJ 08873
(201) 873-2212

---

(1) A residential program using many progressive techniques, including dietary programs and nutritional consultation.

# 16

# Eye Problems

Vision problems often go undetected, even after checkups. For example, during a typical eye examination optometrists may not specifically check for:

- Inaccurate eye movements (ocular motility).
- Unstable eye teaming (binocularity).
- Unstable eye-hand coordination.
- Instability in visual discrimination, visual imagery, and visualization.

Unless such conditions are diagnosed and treated, you may suffer from eye strain, tension, or tired eyes, or you may fall asleep while reading. In children, such conditions can be the cause of hyperactivity or learning disabilities.

## Learn to Take Care of Your Eyes

According to Dr. Marc Grossman, an optometrist and director of the Rye Learning Center in Rye, New York, you should follow these basic guidelines for visual hygiene [from *Whole Life Times*, July/August 1984, p. 10]:

- Give your eyes a break every 20 minutes. Look out the window or simply look away in the distance. In other words, change your focus.
- If you work at a desk, make sure it is slanted upward about 20 degrees, so that material will be parallel to your face. In this way, reading materials will be easier to read.
- Do not stare endlessly at one thing. Glance about and look around you.

- Keep reading materials at an appropriate distance.

These guidelines are just as helpful if you work at a computer terminal.

## For Your Information

If you need to locate a nearby behavioral optometrist who can test your eye movement, call the Optometric Extension Program at 1-800-423-4111. Ask for a doctor who can perform all the aforementioned tests.

# 17

# Fatigue

Fatigue is one of the primary symptoms in thousands of disorders, such as:

- Allergies, including chronic low-grade allergies
- Food-sensitivity reactions
- Hypoglycemia (low blood sugar)
- Low thyroid function
- Anemia
- Poor nutrient absorption
- Structural misalignment of the musculoskeletal system
- Dehydration
- Specific vitamin and mineral deficiencies, for example, deficiencies of magnesium, potassium, and the B vitamins.
- Epstein-Barr virus

Unless your specific condition has been diagnosed professionally, follow the general nutritional recommendations given in this book, as well as the following specific suggestions.

## Use Supplements to Combat Fatigue

If you suffer from fatigue, consider the following supplements:

- Magnesium deficiency is a common cause of fatigue, and magnesium supplementation is therefore highly recommended. In addition, magnesium taken together with potassium has been shown to relieve fatigue.

- Vitamin $B_{12}$ injections can eliminate fatigue caused by poor nutrition.
- Vitamin C is also helpful.
- For women, these supplements are especially helpful: folate, iron, and vitamin $B_{12}$.

## Amino Acid Therapy

If you feel muscular weakness, or if minor exertion causes fatigue, use carnitine. Carnitine is an amino acid that promotes fatty-acid oxidation, which is a major source of energy for your tissues.

## Herbs That Combat Fatigue

To combat fatigue, include such herbs as fo ti, ginseng root, gotu-kola, tincture of capsicum, licorice root, cayenne, garlic, and American centaury in your diet.

For excessive fatigue, avoid herbs that are high in caffeine, for example, guarana and kola nut (bissy nut).

## Homeopathy

Here are some specific remedies to consider:

- For drowsiness: *Cocculus indicus*.
- For tiredness: Phosphoric acid and *Helonia dioca*.
- For lack of energy: Ignatia.
- For exhaustion and fatigue: Zincum met.

## Tissue Salts

Also useful in conditions of fatigue is the tissue salt potassium phosphate 6X.

## Exercise

Regular exercise can clear up many cases of fatigue. To call up the body's reserve fuel supply, *exercise*. It's more effective than eating chocolate or some other sugary snack as a fuel supply!

# 18

## Gallbladder Problems

The most common gallbladder problems concern *gallstones*. Gallstones are composed of cholesterol, which occurs naturally in the bile. When the bile is supersaturated with cholesterol—that is, when it contains more cholesterol than it can store in solution—gallstones begin to form.

### How Good Nutrition Can Help

You can help avoid gallstones by following these nutritional recommendations:

• Follow a modified raw food diet. (See page 23 for information on a modified raw food diet.)

• Become a vegetarian. Studies show that vegetarians have lower rates of gallbladder diseases than nonvegetarians.

• Take at least 2 tablespoons of raw millers bran or oat bran daily. Including at least 50 grams of fiber in your diet each day will help dilute bile acids. Fiber slows down and may even prevent gallstone formation. Raw bran and soybeans help reduce the level of cholesterol saturation in the bile.

• Take vitamin $B_6$ together with corn oil. Studies in Austria show that when these two substances are taken together, they help increase the ability of the bile to dissolve cholesterol. [*Acta Chicurgica Austriaca*, Vol. 8, No. 4, 1976.]

• Avoid whole-milk products. Casein, an animal protein found chiefly in milk products, may increase cholesterol buildup.

- Avoid cold breakfast cereals and granolas (even whole-grain granolas, because oil is often added to granolas).
- Take amino acid supplements. The amino acid methione helps the gallbladder to function normally. Methione is most effective when taken with vitamin $B_6$.

## Juice Therapy

Juice therapy can be very effective in helping to keep your gallbladder functioning properly.

- Drink 3 pints daily of Juice Therapy Formula #6. See the Appendix.
- Squeeze one fresh lemon and add the juice of 6 ounces of hot distilled water. Each day, drink 6 to 10 glasses of this mixture.

## Herbal Remedies

For general gallbladder problems, use the following herbs: agrimony, cascara sagrada, comfrey, mandrake, parsley, wild yam, yellow dock and dandelion.

One folk remedy recommends taking at least two tablespoons of raw millers bran or oat bran (at least 50 grams of dietary fiber) daily.

## Aroma Therapy

Here are two aroma therapies you might try:

- For producing and evacuating bile: Essence of rosemary (rosemary oil).
- For an inflamed gallbladder: Essence of rosemary and oil of pine.

## Massaging Your Gallbladder

To energize your gallbladder, follow these steps:

Stand with your spine straight. Inhale slowly. Hold your breath to a count of 10. Using a kneading action, massage downward in the area of your gallbladder—that is, on the right side of your abdomen, just below the breast.

## Acupressure

Use circular rhythmic pressure in the area of the gallbladder. See Appendix.

## Homeopathy

Homeopathy remedies include podophyllum 3X and celidonium 2X. For gallbladder problems accompanied by fever, take aconitum 4X with the tissue salt phosphate of iron.

# 19

# Gynecological Disorders

Many of the disorders specific to women respond very well to natural healing techniques. Let's look more closely at some of the most common of these gynecological conditions:

*Amenorrhea (Absence of Menses).* The absence of menses may be caused by many different factors. Two common causes are (1) stress and (2) a low percentage of body fat. Ballet dancers, fashion models, and athletes often have very low body-fat levels and therefore tend to suffer from this condition more often than others.

*Menorrhagia (Excess Menstrual Discharge).* Excessive menstrual discharge can contribute to iron deficiency anemia and therefore to fatigue.

*Fibrocystic Breast Disease.* This noncancerous condition is characterized by a tenderness as well as lumps in the breast. Both symptoms are sometimes constant and are generally most prominent one or two weeks prior to menstruation. In the Western Hemisphere, the symptoms are more common between December and May, when the ovaries are more active.

Fibrocystic breast disease may be caused by thyroid deficiency, foods, and drugs that contain methyl-xanthines (caffeine is the best-known chemical in this group).

Women who have fibrocystic breast disease should have exams frequently because they are 2 to 8 times more likely to develop breast cancer.

*Premenstrual Syndrome (PMS).* About 10 days before menstruation begins, the symptoms of PMS begin to appear. These symptoms may include:

| Anxiety | Clumsiness | Craving for salty |
| Fatigue | Difficulty concentrating | or sweet foods |
| Crying for no | Headache | Depression |
| apparent reason | Abdominal bloating | Insomnia |
| Mood swings | Weight gain | Breast tenderness |
| Panic attacks | Increased appetite | |

Many nurses and healers who have worked with PMS patients claim that over two-thirds of these women have difficulty metabolizing simple carbohydrates. Many of their symptoms mimic those of hypoglycemia, including a craving for sweets.

One explanation is that some of the hormones that are secreted during ovulation may increase the breakdown of sugar and the retention of fluids. The drop in the blood-sugar level then sends this signal to the brain: "I need something sweet."

As a result, the diet recommended in PMS cases is identical to the diet recommended in hypoglycemia: a lactovegetarian diet. This diet will be discussed later in this section.

*Trichomoniasis.* This condition is generally transmitted sexually, but it may be spread (1) by improperly wiping the anus or (2) in swimming pools. Trichomoniasis is more common among heavy smokers.

*Vaginitis.* An inflammation of the vagina, vaginitis is characterized by an abnormal yellow or white discharge. The symptoms may include soreness, burning, and itching. Vaginitis may be caused by a yeast infection or by bacteria, intestinal worms, or a vitamin B deficiency.

## How Nutrition Can Help

Good nutrition can help you relieve some of the disorders discussed earlier.

*Anemia.* For anemia associated with excess menstrual discharge, eat foods that are high in iron: fresh peaches, dried fruits, and green leafy vegetables.

*Premenstrual Syndrome.* To relieve the symptoms of PMS, follow a lactovegetarian diet:

1. Eat small meals of complex carbohydrates, with moderate amounts of fat and protein.

2. Reduce your intake of salt, refined carbohydrates, concentrated sugars, and dairy products. Dairy products may interfere with the absorption of magnesium.

3. Avoid nervous-system stimulants such as coffee, tea, alcohol, tobacco, and chocolate, for example. These stimulants can upset your blood-sugar balance.

4. Eat diuretic foods: watermelon, cucumbers, parsley, and asparagus.

5. Eat plenty of green leafy vegetables.

*Amenorrhea.* Try to gain weight. Increase your caloric intake from quality food sources. Even gaining just a few pounds can bring on normal menstruation.

*Fibrocystic Breast Disease.* Stop drinking all caffeinated beverages: coffee, tea (except caffeine-free herbal teas), and cocoa, and stop eating and drinking chocolate products.

## Amino Acid Supplementation

Women who suffer from premenstrual depression should try L-Tryptophan, which has been very helpful in fighting depression.

## Use Supplementation for Specific Disorders

Note which supplements are recommended for specific disorders:

*Fibrocystic Breast Disease.* Take 600 to 800 iu of vitamin E for at least three months, and have your blood pressure checked to monitor any side effects.

*Menorrhagia.* To reduce heavy menstrual bleeding, add vitamin A and bioflavonoids to your daily intake of supplements. For the anemia that sometimes accompanies menorrhagia, take iron, folic acid, and vitamin $B_{12}$.

*Vaginitis and Urethritis.* Take acidophilus to treat the symptoms of vaginitis or urethritis. If taking acidophilus orally does not prove effective, then prepare an acidophilus douche by mixing the acidophilus in sterile water. This douche should kill the organisms that are causing the problem.

*Irregular Menstruation.* Take vitamin $B_{12}$.

*Premenstrual Syndrome (PMS).* For PMS, follow these recommendations:

1. Take calcium and magnesium to reduce cramps. PMS symptoms often indicate a magnesium deficiency, and the calcium helps to lower the blood pressure if you have hypertension.

2. Take 2,000 milligrams of vitamin C three times a day.

3. Take gamma-linoleic acid (GLA), which is found in evening primrose oil. GLA is essential for manufacturing prostoglandins, which are usually deficient in women who have PMS.

4. Take vitamin $B_6$. Vitamin $B_6$ is very useful in many different gynecological disorders, especially in PMS cases. According to reports, vitamin $B_6$ clears up premenstrual acne; relieves anxiety and depression associated with synthetic estrogen therapy; corrects biochemical abnormalities caused by estrogen; prevents and controls various problems associated with pregnancy, including edema and toxemia; and prevents or reduces premenstrual bloating (fluid retention).

5. Take vitamin E to reduce breast tenderness.

## Juice Therapy Can Be Very Helpful

Try the following recommendations:

*For Amenorrhea:* Drink Juice Therapy Formula #15. See Appendix.

*For General Menstrual Problems:* Try a combination of beet, carrot, and fennel juices. Drink dark fruit juices—grape, prune, cherry, and black currant.

*For Premenstrual Syndrome (PMS):* Drink the juices of watermelon, cucumber, asparagus, and parsley.

*For Vaginal Infections:* Add 2 teaspoons of liquid chlorophyll to each serving of carrot juice three times a day.

## Use Herbs for Relief

For relief from general gynecological disorders, try this herbal formula. Prepare a tea using: unicorn root, life root, black cohash, pleurisy root, and fenugreek seed.

Other herbs that are very useful for general gynecological problems are:

| | |
|---|---|
| White willow bark | Fo ti |
| Dong quai | Uva ursi |
| Crampbark | Parsley |
| Red raspberry | Blessed thistle |
| Yarrow | Squaw vine |

Now here are some specific herbal remedies you may want to try:

*For Menstrual Cramps:* Wormwood, pennyroyal, parsley, and ginger.

*For Irregular Menstruation:* Take one cup of lady's mantle tea for three days, then change to one cup of shepherd's purse tea for the next three days. Parsley and Queen Anne's lace (wild carrot) will increase menstrual flow when the irregular menstruation is also abnormally light.

*For Heavy Menstrual Bleeding:* Capsicum, oak bark, cranesbill, white pine bark, yarrow, amaranth, and lady's mantle.

*For Obstructed or Delayed Menstruation:* Motherwort, garlic, and ginger. Women of the Menominee tribe used white cedar bark to bring on menstruation. Cherokee women used skullcap tea.

*For Premenstrual Syndrome:* Cornsilk and parsley to reduce swelling.

NOTE: Pennyroyal, tansey, black cohash, and blue cohash may cause problems if used in excess. Use these herbs carefully.

## Aroma Therapy

Therapies for specific gynecological problems are:

*For Amenorrhea:* Essence of chamomile, cypress, origanum, peppermint, sage, and thyme.

*For Difficulty in Menstruation:* Essence of caraway, juniper, and lavender.

*For Difficult or Painful Menstruation (Dysmenorrhea):* Essence of aniseed, cajeput, chamomile, cypress, juniper, peppermint, rosemary, sage, and tarragon.

*For Irregular Menstruation:* Essence of fennel, sage, lavender, nutmeg, and peppermint.

*For Vaginal Discharge:* Essence of hyssop, lavender, juniper, rosemary, sage, thyme, originum, and terebinth.

*For General Ovarian Problems:* Essence of cypress and sage.

*For Uterine Hemorrhaging (Metrorrhagia):* Essence of cinnamon, cypress, geranium, juniper, and terebinth.

## Acupressure and Massage

Try a gentle rocking and kneading of the abdomen for cramps. Also for cramps, use circular rhythmic pressure as charted on page 245.

## Exercise for Relief From Cramps

To reduce the discomfort of cramps, try the exercises described on page 164.

In addition, aerobic exercise and yoga are helpful in PMS conditions.

## Hydrotherapy

For relief from menstrual cramps, try a sitz bath using yarrow, chamomile, or juniper at body temperature. Also try a sauna or a steam bath for relief.

## Your Emotional Health Contributes!

As with all physical disorders, gynecological conditions, too, are affected by your personal emotional well-being. Use the various techniques described throughout this book to learn how to control the stress around you and to keep a healthy, positive attitude toward yourself and your life.

## Homeopathy

Try these homeopathy remedies:

- For irritability and moodiness: chamomile.
- For pain: belladonna.
- For delayed or obstructed menses: pulsatilla.
- For back pain during menstruation: pulsatilla.
- For general menstrual pain: caulophyllum viburnum.

## Tissue Salts

Use the following tissue salts for the specific conditions noted.

- For cramps: magnesium phosphate 6X.
- For difficult or painful menstruation: magnesium phosphate.
- For vaginal discharge: calcium phosphate. For a milky-white discharge, use potassium chloride.
- For menstrual cramps: combine calcium phosphate, potassium chloride, potassium phosphate, and magnesium phosphate.
- For excess menstrual discharge: silica.

## Tips to Remember

These related facts and recommendations will also be of interest to you:

*Smoking.* Did you know that smoking can aggravate menstrual difficulties? Now you have yet another reason to stop smoking!

*Acupuncture.* According to Dr. Joseph Helms of the Kaiser Permanente Medical Center in Oakland, California, acupuncture can effectively treat menstrual cramps and some of the symptoms of PMS.

*Mastitis.* In the case of mastitis (breast inflammation), stop breast-feeding immediately. Take hot baths. Wear a bra—even while sleeping—but not too tightly, and use lanolin or vitamin A and D on cracked nipples.

*Vaginal Infection (Vaginitis) and Cystitis.* To reduce your chances of getting these disorders, remember to:

- Change tampons often, and douche after each menstrual period to remove any tampon fibers.

• Dry yourself extra carefully after bathing. Careful drying is more effective than douching in preventing vaginal odors.

• Avoid using soaps that may irritate, vaginal deodorants, perfumed vaginal sprays, colored toilet tissue, and bubble bath products. You can create your own bubble baths using plain soap.

• Wear only cotton underwear. Synthetic fabrics retain heat and moisture, which support bacteria growth. Also, be sure to buy cool, loose underwear (as well as pants and pantyhose), not too tight-fitting.

• If necessary, use a lubricant during intercourse. Also, have your partner wear a condom for added protection.

• After a bowel movement, prevent bacteria from entering the vagina by carefully wiping the anus in a front-to-back motion.

• Cut out refined carbohydrates (white rice; white, refined flour products; white and brown sugars).

• Use acidophilus and eat yogurt on a daily basis.

• Avoid antibiotics unless absolutely necessary.

*Menstrual Irregularities.* Some menstrual problems may result when you are not exposed to light during a certain time of your menstrual cycle. To avoid this possibility, simply keep a small nightlight (say, a 25-watt bulb) on in your bedroom all evening on the 14th through the 17th nights after the beginning of your menstrual period. The light must merely be in the room, it does not need to be directly over you.

This technique has proved positive in about 40 percent of the cases in which it was tried.

*Premenstrual Syndrome.* Herbal diuretics and sedatives can also be very helpful in PMS conditions.

*Douching.* Except in special cases (for example, for medical reasons and in those instances discussed in this section), vaginal douching should be discouraged for several reasons:

• Douching upsets the natural mucus present in the vagina.

• Perfumed and so-called ''flavored'' douches, vaginal deodorants, and similar products contain chemicals that can cause allergic reactions.

• Solutions that are not diluted properly can damage sensitive vaginal tissue.

If you must douche to treat a vaginal disorder, never do so during menses.

Note that simply wiping the lips will sufficiently clean the area. If you prefer, you can wipe with a skin cleanser specifically made for sensitive skin. [Emrika Padus, *The Women's Encyclopedia of Health & Natural Healing*, Rodale Press, Emmaus, Pennsylvania, 1981, pp. 218–219.]

*Sitz Baths.* As an alternative to douching, make a hot sitz bath. Crush a fresh clove of garlic in the sitz bath. The garlic oil, which is released in the hot water, produces positive results in the treatment of vaginal infections, especially trichomaniasis. [Emrika Padus, *The Women's Encyclopedia of Health & Natural Healing*, Rodale Press, Emmaus, Pennsylvania, 1981, pp. 296.]

## For More Information

These resources may be valuable if you need further information:

National PMS Society          Premenstrual Syndrome Action
P.O. Box 11467                P.O. Box 9326
Durham, NC 27703              Madison, WI 53715

# 20

# Headaches

Perhaps the most common ailment that people mention is the *headache*. What causes a headache?

Among the hundreds of possible causes of headaches, the most prevalent are these:

• Premenstrual Syndrome (see "Gynecological Disorders" for more information on PMS)
• Excessive salt intake
• Dehydration
• Wheat sensitivity
• Eating very cold food (for example, ice cream)
• Hangovers (that is, the aftereffect of drinking alcohol)
• A radical change in sleeping patterns or relaxation patterns
• Inhaling noxious fumes
• High blood pressure
• Glaucoma
• Infections
• Sinus disease
• Poor diet
• Eye strain
• Inadequate sleep or excessive sleep
• A blood clot in the brain

- Anxiety
- Depression
- Arthritis
- Allergies
- Hypoglycemia
- Spinal subluxations
- Joint dysfunction
- Narrow-focus syndrome (that is, focusing your eyes too intensely on one subject)
- General structural imbalances (including poor posture)

## Types of Headaches

Let's take a closer look at the types of headaches that are most common:

*Migraine Headaches.* A migraine headache results when an artery in the head dilates. As the artery dilates, it throbs and stretches the vessel wall, and the stretching causes pain. Even before the artery dilates, however, it may constrict or spasm, and these constrictions or spasms are responsible for the symptoms that generally seem unrelated to the headache, such as ringing in the ears, slurred speech, dizziness, and tingling of the skin on one side of the body.

Migraines can be caused by hormonal changes, especially an increase in estrogen. Women who take estrogen supplements or oral contraceptives may experience more migraines than women who do not take hormone-based products.

In addition, migraines can be caused by a number of other factors, such as sensitivity to very bright lights or to sunshine, very cloudy weather conditions, active low-pressure weather, excessive hunger, and some common odors, for example, tobacco smoke, aerosols, paint thinner, and car-exhaust fumes.

*Environmental Headaches.* Environmental headaches include those caused by the sensitivity to certain foods and food additives, especially monosodium glutamate, popularly known as MSG. They also include headaches that result from allergies, functional hypoglycemia, and caffeine withdrawal.

*Muscle Contractions.* This broad category includes headaches caused by daily stress and tension, as well as by contractions in the neck muscles during sexual excitement or orgasm.

Other causes of muscle-contraction headaches are poor posture, temporomandibular joint syndrome (TMJ), which includes bruxism (grinding of the teeth) and poor dental bite, depression, and keeping the neck or head in the same position for an extended period of time (for example while reading or watching television).

Perhaps 90 percent of all headaches are muscle-contraction headaches.

*Cluster Headaches.* A "cluster headache" describes severe headaches that appear in groups of, say, four or more headaches in one day. Each headache may last from 30 minutes to 2 hours. The cluster may recur every day, or it can be weeks or months apart.

Cluster headaches may be caused by hot air or cold wind blowing on the face. They may also be caused by any chemical additive that dilates the blood vessels—nitrates, for example.

Cluster headaches are more common among people who smoke and who drink alcohol.

*Organic Headaches.* Organic headaches may be associated with diseases—brain tumors, herpes zoster, inflammation of the blood vessels in the temple, and sinus infections.

*Posttraumatic Headaches.* Headaches that result from surgery or from an injury are called *posttraumatic* headaches.

*Exertional Headaches.* This is a headache that results from coughing, sneezing, or some other form of physical exertion or strain. Exertional headaches are usually harmless, but they are sometimes associated with brain disease. Therefore, they should be checked by a professional to make sure that there is no serious underlying cause.

## How Nutrition Can Help You Stop Headaches

Proper nutrition can be very effective in preventing headaches, as well as in alleviating a headache once it begins. Here are some general guidelines for prevention of, as well as relief from, headaches.

### Prevention

• Eliminate *slowly* any caffeinated beverages you generally drink—coffee, cola drinks, and tea. Cut them out gradually and you will avoid possible headaches resulting from the withdrawal process, especially if you have been drinking these beverages for a long time. Because most herbal teas contain no caffeine, they serve as excellent substitutes.

• Avoid eating foods with MSG. Likewise, avoid nitrates and nitrites, both of which are found in many processed foods such as deli foods and prepackaged sandwich meats (salami, hot dogs, and so on).

### Relief

*Migraines.* Some constituents of foods may create a chemical imbalance that, in turn, may cause the migraine. Therefore, to avoid migraine headaches, be sure not to consume the following:

Alcoholic Products (especially champagne and red wine)

Broad bean pods, fava beans, lima beans, navy beans, and pea pods

Sauerkraut

Papaya products

Brewer's yeast

Canned figs

Aged and sharp cheeses:

| | | |
|---|---|---|
| Swiss | Emmemtaler | Brie |
| Parmesan | Provolone | Cheddar |
| Brick | Blue cheese | Gruyere |
| Camembert | Mozzarella | Stilton |
| Gouda | Romano | Roquefort |

Foods containing cheese (pizza and macaroni, for example)

Dairy products, including yogurt, sour cream, and buttermilk

Other foods to steer clear of include chicken liver, chocolate, citrus fruits, coffee, cola drinks, corn, eggs, garlic, onion, homemade yeast breads, cakes, desserts made from yeast, pickled herring, shellfish, pork, cinnamon, bay leaves, and wheat.

*Hangovers.* Drink tomato juice and plenty of nonalcoholic liquids. Also, eat foods rich in fructose, such as fruit or honey.

*Headaches Caused by Hypoglycemia.* Follow the nutritional suggestions for hypoglycemia (see page 105).

## Supplement Your Diet

Take L-Tryptophan to reduce the pain of migraine headaches.

## Your Daily Supplementation Program

Be sure to include the following in your daily supplementation program:

Vitamin B Complex          Magnesium
Calcium                    L-Tryptophan

## Herbs That Can Help

Here are three herbal formulas that you will find helpful for headaches:

**Formula #1:**

Black cohash          Lobelia
Hops flowers          Skullcap
Valerian root         Wood betany
Cayenne

**Formula #2:**

Black cohash          Basil
Willow bark           Marjoram
Vervain               Rosemary

**Formula #3:**

Rosemary       Chamomile
Comfrey        Lobelia

## Aroma Therapy

Try oils of lavender, lemon, and peppermint. For headaches associated with influenza, use oil of chamomile.

## Acupressure and Massage

You can relieve headache pain in various ways:

1. Press the point at the top side of the hand on the fleshy area between the forefinger and the thumb. Apply pressure to this contact point on both hands.

2. Apply Circular Rhythmic Pressure.

3. Have chiropractic adjustments regularly. Chiropractic adjustments or other

physical manipulations are especially recommended when the cause of headaches cannot be tied to medical problems, nutritional factors, or allergies.

Acupuncture—particularly acupuncture of the ear—is also effective in relieving all kinds of headaches, especially migraine headaches.

## Exercise As a Cure

There are a number of ways in which you can reduce migraine pain—or better yet, help prevent migraines from occurring.

*Aerobic Exercises.* According to reports, migraine sufferers who began an aerobic-exercise program had half as many headaches as they had before starting the program. People involved in the study, walked or ran 30 minutes a day at least three times a week. If you suffer from migraine headaches and do not exercise regularly, you now have an added incentive to exercise!

*Neck-Rolling Exercises.* To improve your circulation and reduce congestion in the neck and the head, do neck-rolling exercises.

*Breathing Exercises.* Breathe into a bag, and then *re*breathe the exhaled air from the bag. Repeat this procedure for 15 to 20 minutes for relief from migraine headaches.

## Hydrotherapy for Migraines

If you suffer from migraine headaches, try one of these hydrotherapy techniques:

1. Alternate taking cold and hot showers—cold first, then hot.
2. Apply an onion or a horseradish poultice to the nape of your neck. The poultice will draw blood pressure away from the neck. [A. Vogel, *Swiss Nature Doctor*, Switzerland, 1980.]
3. Apply a cabbage compress above the eyes.

## Homeopathy

Among the homeopathy remedies that are most effective are these:
*For General Headaches:* Salix nig and coffea.
*For Headache Accompanied by Sore Muscles:* Belladonna.

## Tissue Salts

Try these tissue salts for headache relief:
*For General Headaches:* Phosphate of iron 6X or potassium phosphate 6X.
*For Migraine and Tension Headaches:* Combine potassium phosphate, magnesium phosphate, sodium chloride, and silicic oxide.
*For Headaches Accompanied by Muscle Cramps:* Magnesium phosphate.

## Tips to Remember

*Environmental Headaches.* To help avoid environmental headaches, follow the nutritional recommendations in the section on "Allergies."

*Cluster Headaches.* Oxygen therapy is the most effective natural healing technique for cluster headaches. Unfortunately, it is impractical to have oxygen at hand all the time. Therefore, this therapy is best employed by people who suffer cluster attacks in the evenings because they can keep oxygen at their bedsides.

*Muscle Contractions and Posttraumatic Headaches.* Massage and biofeedback are both preventives and healing tools for muscle contractions.

For temporomandibular joint (TMJ) problems, see a chiropractor, osteopath, dentist, or medical doctor for special exercises, manipulations, or adjustments. (Also see Dental and Oral Problems.) You may benefit from a special appliance such as a bite plate or a dental implant.

*Organic Headaches.* In the case of organic headaches, the "cure" is to treat the disease that causes the headaches, rather than the symptoms themselves.

## For Your Information

For an updated list of headache specialists and clinics throughout the United States, contact:

National Migraine Foundation
5214 N. Western Avenue
Chicago, IL 60625
(312) 878-7715

# 21

# Herpes

New detection methods show that as much as one quarter of the American population may have genital herpes. Yet the majority of the people who have this viral infection are unaware of it; for one reason, because they experience no symptoms. Others who have herpes experience either occasional blisters or constant, painful blisters.

## What is Herpes?

Herpes is a virus that is passed from infected carriers to others through physical contact—by touching mucous membranes or cuts, for example. The herpes virus belongs to the same family as chicken pox.

Actually, there are *two* herpes viruses, called "simplex I" and "simplex II."

Herpes *simplex I* is the virus that causes cold sores and blisters in the mouth. This virus usually burrows into the nerve cells near the brain.

Herpes *simplex II* generally infects the genital area. The most common symptoms are lesions and blisters, but flu-like symptoms and headaches may also occur. Whereas simplex I burrows near the brain, simplex II invades the spinal cord.

Although neither of these virus infections is life-threatening, a herpes infection is a lifelong disease: There is no known cure for herpes.

## A Nutritional Approach to Herpes Control

In both cases, there will be active and dormant periods. Research shows that herpes attacks may be suppressed when the patient's intake of two amino acids is carefully maintained. The amino acids are arginine and lysine, and they must be taken in a 1:1 ratio, that is, in equal amounts.

## Amino Acid Therapy

The herpes simplex virus needs arginine to reproduce, and lysine is antagonistic to arginine. Lysine, therefore, can work magically on herpes symptoms. Lysine can stop herpes pain overnight, speed up recovery from herpes symptoms, stop the spread of herpes lesions, and promote healing.

Further, when lysine was taken in maintenance dosages, it prevented herpes symptoms from recurring. [Carlton Fredericks, "Hotline to Health," *Prevention Magazine*, XXXII, January, 1980, p. 42.]

## Your Supplementation Program

Here is a daily supplementation program that will help:

Lysine (1,200 milligrams)        Vitamin A
Zinc                             Vitamin B complex
Calcium

## Herbal Therapy

Herbs are particularly useful for reducing the blisters that occur in herpes conditions:

Chaparral leaves                             *Echinacea purpurea*
Sage                                         Sarsaparilla root
*Tragancantha astragulus*                    Black walnut
Dehydrated juice from young barley plants    Oregon grape root
Yellow dock root

The Green Magma brand of dehydrated juice from young barley plants is available in most health food stores.

## Aroma Therapy

Try oil of geranium and oil of lemon for relief from herpes symptoms.

## Control Your Emotions

As we have noted throughout this book, in many physical conditions the patient's emotional approach to life is a very important factor, and herpes is no exception. The intensity and frequency of herpes eruptions is strongly affected by stress and tension.

To help control herpes symptoms, reduce the level of stress in your life. Add humor to your everyday routine. Try visualization, biofeedback, meditation, and yoga in an effort to reduce tension and stress.

## Also of Interest

A topical cream made from lysine and zinc oxide has been reported to be effective in healing eruptions of genital herpes.

# 22

# Hypertension

The cause of hypertension, which is an abnormal rise in blood pressure, is not clearly known. Among the factors that are most likely to contribute are:

- Undetected allergies
- Family history
- Dietary habits
- Stress
- Poor, stressful communication skills (People who have very rapid, aggressive speech patterns generally have higher blood pressure than people who speak slowly and without stress.)
- Impaired kidney function
- Glandular problems
- Defective calcium metabolism
- Arteriosclerosis

Some people who suffer from very high blood pressure may have no symptoms; others, however, may experience a variety of symptoms, including headaches, insomnia, edema, shortness of breath, blurred vision, nosebleeds, nervousness, or irritability.

Hypertension is a very serious condition because it can lead to kidney failure, strokes, and heart conditions.

## Black Americans Are Especially Susceptible

The incidence of hypertension among Black Americans is unusually high. Why are Black Americans twice as likely to suffer from hypertension than non-Black Americans?

The answer appears to be genetic predisposition. Black Americans have an unusual ability to retain salt, a characteristic that is beneficial to people who have little salt in their diets and who live in exceptionally hot climates, but it is definitely harmful in our American culture.

As we already mentioned, hypertension can lead to kidney failure, strokes, and heart conditions. Black Americans, therefore, are more likely to suffer from these results of hypertension, according to a study by Dr. Clarence Grim of the Los Angeles Postgraduate School of Medicine. ["Blacks' Hypertension and Salt Link," *New York Times*, August 19, 1986.]

## Nutritional Guidelines

You can control—better yet, *avoid*—hypertension if you are careful.

*Avoid Caffeinated Beverages.* The first step toward lowering your chances of developing hypertension is to stop drinking caffeinated beverages. Studies show that even a few cups of coffee (or its equivalent) can raise your diastolic blood pressure an average of 14 percent *within one hour*.

*Try the Watermelon Diet.* Try a diet of only watermelon for one week. NOTE: Do not attempt this diet if you have diabetes or hypoglycemia.

*Limit Your Sodium Intake.* Sodium is an essential nutrient, but excessive amounts of sodium may contribute to high blood pressure. For one thing, sodium causes fluid retention, and excess fluid adds stress to the heart and the circulatory system.

One teaspoon of table salt contains about 2,000 mg of sodium. According to the National Research Council, an adult can safely take about 1,100 to 3,300 mg of sodium daily. (Some estimates show that the average American adult now consumes from 2,300 to 6,900 mg of sodium daily!). Thus, you must monitor your sodium intake carefully, not an easy chore, because sodium may be scattered throughout your diet.

Do you add salt to your foods at the table? If salt has been added to your foods during the processing or during the cooking, then you are adding *additional* salt. To eliminate salt as a food additive, avoid these foods:

| | |
|---|---|
| Baking soda and baking powder | Salty fish |
| Sodium nitrate and sodium nitrite | Most snack foods, including |
| Monosodium glutamate (MSG) |    desserts |
| Most cheeses (unless labeled "Salt-Free") | Foods containing soy sauce |
| Meat (especially processed meat) | Tamarai |
| Pickles | Shoyu |
| Olives | Salt brine |

Your first step? Read the labels on all food packages. Labels that claim "low sodium" will specify the sodium content. Generally, however, remember that unprocessed, fresh foods have much less sodium than processed, packaged foods.

To reduce the sodium intake at mealtime, learn to use lemon juice, apple cider vinegar, cayenne pepper, and onion or garlic powder instead of prepared sauces and high-salt condiments. And when you're in a restaurant, look for the low-sodium selections on the menu!

*Break the sugar habit.* Sugar may stop the body from eliminating sodium. Thus sugar increases your sodium retention and, as a result, your blood pressure. If you have hypertension, eliminate refined sugar from your diet.

*Follow a raw vegetarian diet.* Studies show that hypertensive people who switched to low-fat vegetarian diets radically lowered their blood pressure. In fact, reducing your intake of fats may be even more effective for lowering your blood pressure than reducing your salt intake.

Perhaps the high potassium content of the foods in a raw food diet is responsible. Foods that are high in potassium are recommended for lowering blood pressure:

| | | |
|---|---|---|
| Orange juice | Apricots | Avocados |
| Potatoes | Lima beans | Tomatoes |
| Squash | Bananas | Peaches |

*Increase Your Calcium Intake.* An inadequate intake of calcium may contribute to hypertension. Recent studies show that Blacks and the elderly—two groups that have higher risks of hypertension—often have calcium deficiencies.

Among the foods that are high in calcium are yogurt, chickpeas, and tofu.

*Eat Onions.* Onions contain prostaglandin-Al, a hormone-like chemical that lowers blood pressure.

## The Role of Supplements

Studies have shown that you can lower not only your blood pressure but also your cholesterol and triglyceride levels by proper diet, a diet that includes the essential fatty acids (EFAs), which are found in certain vegetable oils.

Two important contributors to the supplementation program for lowering blood pressure are the amino acids GABA (gamma-aminobutryic acid) and proline.

## Juice Therapy

Many healers consider juice fasting *the* most efficient method for lowering systolic pressure. For best results, use Juice Therapy Formula #12 (see Appendix) for two to four weeks. If this is too concentrated a time period, try several one-week-long fasts over a period of about six months.

Besides Juice Therapy Formula #12, you can use all citrus juices such as watermelon, beet, cranberry (unsweetened), spinach, and grape.

## Herbal Remedies

Try hawthorn, wild cherry bark and valerian to help lower your blood pressure. On the other hand, avoid using strong spices and herbs such as mustard, black and white pepper, ginger, and nutmeg.

## Aroma Therapy

Several essences are known to be effective in lowering blood pressure:

- Essence of calamus is believed to reduce blood pressure by dilating the splenic vessels.

• Essence of hyssop initially increases, but then shortly afterward decreases, blood pressure.

• Essences of garlic, lavender, lemon, marjoram, and ylang-ylang are also effective.

## Acupressure and Massage

Apply Deep Rhythmic Pressure (see Appendix). Also, be sure to dry brush massage daily.

## Emotional Factors

Stress, worry, anxiety, tension—all contribute to hypertension. If you are to control your blood pressure, a good starting point is to try to control your emotional reactions to your surroundings.

## Exercise

Following an aerobic-exercise program regularly is extremely valuable in reducing hypertension.

## Lower Blood Pressure Through Natural Healing

James R., a computer programmer, always felt fine, had plenty of energy, and slept very well, despite the fact that he led a sedentary life and ate plenty of red meat and greasy, fatty foods.

One day, during a routine company physical, the examining doctor checked James' blood pressure. Knowing that James reported no symptoms to indicate high blood pressure, the doctor was really surprised to find James' pressure at 160/120. In fact, the doctor decided to repeat the test, just to make sure that the first results weren't affected by any outside causes. But the results were the same: 160/120.

Because James was allergic to the medication that the doctor wanted to prescribe, James went to a nutritionist instead, and that's how he began a natural healing program for lowering his blood pressure.

• He began following a controlled-calorie, low-sodium, lactovegetarian diet: no red meat, no fatty foods, no hot or spicy foods; plenty of fresh garlic and onion; a combination of fresh-pressed juices three times a day, including breakfast: 6 oz. cucumber, 4 oz. carrot, and 2 oz. parsley; and supplements of potassium and vitamin $B_6$.

• He began walking 40 minutes every day.

• He watched a visualization tape daily to reduce on-the-job stress.

In just six weeks, James was able to lower his blood pressure from 160/120 to an acceptable 120/80, thanks to this natural healing program.

# 23

# Hypoglycemia

Hypoglycemia is the subject of much controversy. Because many of the symptoms of hypoglycemia are mental or emotional, allopathic physicians generally do not take hypoglycemia seriously. In fact, most consider it a condition that really exists only "in the patient's head."

On the other hand, natural healers certainly do see hypoglycemia as "real." However, they tend to agree that hypoglycemia is not a disease but a symptom of other physical problems. As a result, they try to find and treat the cause of the problem.

Let's take a closer look at the two different types of hypoglycemia, *fasting hypoglycemia* and *functional hypoglycemia*.

## Fasting Hypoglycemia

Of all the people who have hypoglycemia, about 30 percent suffer from *fasting hypoglycemia*, a condition that can result from a number of rare conditions, such as:

- Liver disease
- Adrenal or pituitary insufficiency
- Tumors (especially in the pancreas)
- Excessive alcohol consumption by diabetics
- An excessive dose of insulin or of other antidiabetic substances by diabetics

Other factors may also lead to fasting hypoglycemia:

| | |
|---|---|
| Inability to cope with stress | Lack of sunlight |
| Lack of exercise | Overeating refined foods and sugars |
| Poor dietary habits | Food allergies |
| Poor absorption of nutrients | Weak adrenal glands |
| Insufficient stomach acid | (hypoadrenocorticism) |

## Functional Hypoglycemia

This is the type of hypoglycemia that orthodox doctors question. To the natural healer, functional hypoglycemia is not only real but a serious threat to normal everyday life.

The symptoms of functional hypoglycemia are related to meals; *what* the patient eats and *when* he or she eats. In the early stages of functional hypoglycemia, the patient may feel light-headedness at midmorning and in late afternoon. But in later stages, the patient may experience many other symptoms, including:

| | |
|---|---|
| Fatigue or exhaustion | Hunger |
| Headaches | Dizziness |
| Heart palpitations | Weak spells |
| Muscular aches or twitches | Fainting |
| Skin-tingling sensation | Double or blurred vision |
| Excessive sweating | Cold hands or feet |
| Gasping for breath | Craving for sugar |
| Trembling | Chronic indigestion and nausea |

In addition to all the above physical symptoms, the patient may also experience a variety of psychological symptoms, such as confusion, absent-mindedness, loss of memory, restlessness and depression.

## A Nutritional Approach to Treating Hypoglycemia

To control hypoglycemia, most natural healers recommend following this two-step approach:

1. Follow a diet high in complex carbohydrates and moderate in protein, but be sure to test how each individual carbohydrate food affects you. Some individuals can experience rapid drops in their blood-sugar levels from certain seemingly harmless carbohydrates.

2. Eat six or more small meals a day, rather than just a few large meals. This slowly and regularly releases nutrients and sugars into your bloodstream rather than all at once.

In addition to following these two major steps, be sure to:

*Control Your Sodium Intake.* Use only as much salt as you need for nutritional purposes, *and no more*. Excessive salt consumption may cause a loss of blood potassium and a drop in the blood-sugar level.

*Eat Breakfast Regularly.* Eat breakfast regularly to help you normalize your blood-sugar levels. Eat whole-grain cereals with soy milk or goat's milk.

*Eat Vegetables and Beans.* Eat those carbohydrates that are slowly absorbed— for example, vegetables, beans, whole-grain products, and certain fruits.

*Avoid Fruit Juices.* If you must drink fruit juice, dilute it half and half with distilled water. Likewise, avoid eating large amounts of fruit at one sitting.

*Avoid Caffeine.* Do not drink coffee, tea (except caffeine-free herbal teas), and cocoa products.

*Eliminate Sugars.* Do not use white, brown, or raw sugars or any foods that contain sugars.

## Testing for Hypoglycemia

Careful testing is required to determine whether someone has hypoglycemia.

*Glucose-Tolerance Test.* In the glucose-tolerance test, the patient's blood is taken every 30 minutes for a period of five or six hours. During the process, the patient is also given substances containing glucose. In this way, the patient's ability to maintain a normal blood-sugar level is determined.

The glucose-tolerance test is the most common and the best evaluation tool used to diagnose hypoglycemia.

*Adrenal Gland Function.* To test the adrenal gland function, the patient's urine is collected over a 24-hour period. The urine is then tested for the 30 to 50 hormones that are produced by the adrenal gland.

*RAST Test.* This food-allergy test determines whether allergies are really the cause of the patient's low blood sugar.

## Amino Acid Therapy

Two amino acids that are useful in treating hypoglycemia are alanine and cysteine.

## Supplements That Help

The primary supplements that help control hypoglycemia are:

*Vitamins C and B.* These vitamins assist in normalizing sugar metabolism by increasing the body's tolerance for sugars and carbohydrates.

*Pantothenic Acid, Vitamin B$_6$, and B Complex.* These nutrients strengthen the adrenal gland function.

*Vitamin E.* Vitamin E improves glycogen storage in the muscles and tissues.

## Use Herbs to Control Hypoglycemia

Raw garlic extract, Oregon grape root, licorice root, goldenseal root, uva ursi leaves, mullein leaves, and cayenne are among the herbs that can help you control hypo glycemia.

## A Moody Teenager Becomes Pleasant and Cheerful

Although Susan K. was only 17 years old, she had been plagued by emotional problems for a number of years. She was often irritable and moody. After eating sweets, which she always craved, she had bursts of energy but within an hour she would feel depressed and weak.

When her psychotherapist suggested the possibility that the root of Susan's problems might be a nutritional deficiency or an allergy of some kind, her parents consulted a nutritionally oriented physician. The physician gave Susan a glucose-tolerance test. And then the cause became clear: Susan K. had hypoglycemia.

Could she keep her favorite foods—spaghetti and burgers—in her new diet and still keep her condition under control? She could!

By making the changes suggested in this section, improvement was fast. Within one week, Susan was noticeably less irritable, she had more energy and she was pleasant to be with. On those few occasions when Susan went off her diet and gave in to her cravings for sugar, her emotional swings returned. Susan realizes that she *must* maintain her special diet to keep her hypoglycemia under control.

# 24

# Immune-System Disorders

*Immunity* is the process by which the body resists disease. Essentially a protection system, immunity is really two systems.

The *nonspecific immune system*, the body's first line of defense, protects us from viruses, bacteria, various parasites and fungi. To protect us, this system employs a number of special body cells, compounds, and reactions, including "phagocytes, interferon, lysozyme, iron-binding proteins, fever and a complex set of enzymes called the complement system, which enhances the effectiveness of antibodies and promotes other nonspecific types of resistance." [Jane E. Brody, "Personal Health," *The New York Times*, March 11, 1987, Section C, p. 10.]

The *specific immune system* uses molecules and cells generated by the body's lymphoid organs to attack certain fungal and viral infections. The lymphoid organs include the thymus, spleen, lymph nodes, and bone marrow.

## Breakdowns Lead to Infections

Together, the nonspecific and the specific immune systems make up the army that protects the body from disease. But this defensive army can break down or weaken when under attack, for example, as a result of poor sanitary habits, sexual transmission of immune-weakening disorders (such as AIDS), poor nutritional habits, and negative emotions, particularly depression.

The result of a weakening or a breakdown in the immune system is an *infection*, which is essentially an invasion of the body by a disease-producing organism, usually through the skin or the mucous membrane. The "invaders" may be fungi, parasites, bacteria, viruses, or rickettsiae (microorganisms that are bigger than viruses but smaller than bacteria).

Among the common infectious diseases are:

• Infections of the upper-respiratory tract, such as colds, influenza, sore throats, and laryngitis.

• Ear infections.

• Sinusitis.

• Infections of the mouth, such as gingivitis, periodontitis, stomatitis, molar abscesses, and cold sores.

• Bronchial infections.

• Lung infections, such as pneumonia.

• Cardiovascular infections, such as infective endocarditis, myocarditis, and periocarditis.

• Infections of the nervous system, such as meningitis and encephalitis.

• Infections of the skin and soft tissue, such as impetigo and toxic shock syndrome.

• Gastrointestinal infections, such as diarrhea and food poisoning.

• Infections of the joints and bones, such as infectious arthritis and osteomyelitis.

• Urinary tract infections, such as urethra, prostate gland, bladder, and kidney infections.

• Sexually transmitted diseases, such as gonorrhea, vaginitis, genital herpes, syphilis, and AIDS.

## Fighting Infection Through Good Nutrition

Poor nutrition weakens the immune system and makes you susceptible to infection. Your first step toward developing a solid nutrition program is to avoid all products that contain white flour, white rice, white or brown sugar, and refined products in general. White sugar may actually diminish the body's immune response.

Some general dietary conditions that undermine the immune system are:

• Malnutrition

• Obesity

• A deficiency in EFAs

• Overconsumption of polyunsaturates

• High blood-cholesterol levels

*The Value of a Macrobiotic or a Vegan Diet.* A macrobiotic diet is very effective for healing systemic infection: eat plenty of miso soup, umoboshi plums, and fresh ginger. Also helpful is alternating a vegan diet with juice fasting for one week or two weeks.

For example, for mononucleosis—an infectious disease of the lymph glands accompanied by swollen glands, fever, chills, and sore throat—a lactovegetarian or macrobiotic diet can be very effective. In addition, increasing protein intake helps combat mononucleosis because the protein helps stimulate the formation of antibodies.

## Amino Acid Therapy

A number of amino acids are known to help improve the immune-system response:

- *Arginine* stimulates the immune response by enhancing the body's T cells.
- *Carnitine* is effective in enhancing immune function.
- *L-Cysteine* assists the white blood cells in destroying viruses and bacteria.
- *L-Arginine*, according to some reports, helps to strengthen the immune system by increasing T-cell function and resistance to viruses and bacteria. The effectiveness of this amino acid is increased when it is taken together with vitamins C and $B_1$.
- *L-Ornithine* is even more effective than L-Arginine in improving immune response. Both amino acids are often taken together.

## Supplements That Help

Deficiencies of these nutrients are known to interfere with or undermine the immune response: vitamins A, E, C, and the B vitamins (especially vitamin $B_6$, pantothenic acid, and folic acid), copper, iodine, and selenium.

Note the positive properties of the following supplements in improving immune-system response:

- *Acidophilus* inhibits the growth of toxin-producing microorganisms and produces natural antibiotics.
- *DMG (dimethylglycine)* increases antibody production and generates lymphocytes, which are highly beneficial for anyone with a low-activity immune system response.
- *Lipotropes*—vitamin $B_{12}$, choline, folic acid, and methionine—are essential for synthesizing nucleic acids and forming new body cells.
- *Vitamin A* fights viral infections and increases resistance to disease. In one study, vitamin A supplementation was shown to (1) reduce the number of respiratory infections in children and (2) lessen the severity of the few infections the children did have.

Vitamin A is essential for the division of T cells and B cells, both of which are necessary for proper immune response. But note that excessive amounts of vitamin A can suppress immune response!

- *Vitamin $B_1$*, when taken together with vitamin C, selenium, magnesium, and the amino acid L-Cysteine reduces the negative effects of free radicals and helps strengthen immune-system response.
- Vitamin $B_6$ is required for proper functioning of the epithelial cells of the thymus gland, which is an essential part of the immune system. Vitamin $B_6$ deficiencies have been directly linked with immune-system disorders.
- *Potassium and vitamin C* help compensate for nutritional losses during fevers, which are often associated with infections and immune-system disorders.
- *Zinc* is essential for the proper maintenance of T cells and assists in transporting

and storing vitamin A. Zinc deficiencies have been directly associated with a reduction in cell-mediated immunity and a shrinking of the thymus gland.

• Vitamin C is very important for increasing immune response. It stimulates the production of interferon, a protein that fights viral infection. It can increase the amount of antibodies available to fight off diseases. It increases the production of lymphocytes, and strengthens white blood cells, which seek out and destroy microorganisms.

In very high doses, vitamin C is administered intravenously to treat polio and encephalitis.

• *Selenium* strengthens the immune system by increasing various components of the body's defense system, including B cells and lysozymes.

• *Magnesium* deficiency can reduce your immune response by lowering antibody levels.

## Juice Therapy

The juices listed below are excellent tonics for strengthening the immune system.

| | | |
|---|---|---|
| Carrot | Orange | Green peppers |
| Black currant | Garlic | Watercress |
| Lemon | Beet | Pineapple |

## Include Herbs in Your Program

Among the herbs that help improve immune response are these:

| | | |
|---|---|---|
| *Liquistrum lucidum* | Echinacea | Myrhh |
| Siberian ginseng | Thyme | Goldenseal |
| Propolis | Juniper berries | Cayenne |
| *Astragalus membranaceus* | Chaparral | Osha root |
| *Glycyrrhiza uralensis* | Rosemary | Rose hips |
| Pau d'Arco | Garlic | |

## Aroma Therapy

Essential oils have long been known for their antibacterial activity, perhaps because they stimulate leukocytosis and thus increase the immune response.

Lavender is the most effective essence for increasing leukocytosis. Also helpful are: bergamot, chamomile, thyme, lemon, pine needle, and sandlewood oils.

The most effective oils for topical use are cinnamon, eucalyptus, and origanum. Essences work most effectively—both in aroma therapy and in topical massaging—when they are *not* combined with other oils.

## Acupressure and Massage

Use kneading and circular rhythmic pressure, as seen on the chart in the Appendix.

## Hydrotherapy

Sponge and bathe with cool water. Also, alternate between hot showers and cold showers.

## Visualization and Relaxation

Harvard psychologist Mary Jasnoski studied the effect of relaxation techniques on the immune system. One group of students "imagined their immune systems attacking weak cold and flu viruses" with starting results:

They "were successful in boosting their immune system, hiking up two important types of immune cells—salivary immunoglobin A cells, which battle colds and other upper-respiratory ills, and helper T cells, which spur antibody production." [*New York Sunday News*, September 28, 1986, p. 12.]

# 25

# Irritable Bowel Syndrome (IBS)

Irritable bowel syndrome—"IBS" for short—is the term used to describe a number of gastrointestinal problems, including these three common conditions: nervous diarrhea, spastic colon and mucous colitis.

## Common Symptoms

IBS is really a symptom of some other underlying disorder; it is not a disease in itself. Whatever the cause, the result is that the smooth muscles of the large intestine spasm and cause uneven contractions. The contractions then move any food in the bowel either too quickly (causing diarrhea) or too slowly (causing constipation).

Besides diarrhea and constipation, IBS may exhibit many other possible symptoms, including:

| | |
|---|---|
| Migraine headaches | Abdominal bloating |
| Menstrual cramps | Rectal bleeding |
| Heartburn | Rectal mucous discharge |
| Nausea | |

Initial symptoms generally are seen in people between the ages of 20 and 40.

## Probable Causes

Stress is considered a major factor in IBS conditions, but intolerance of certain foods is probably a greater culprit. Other causes include:

- Antibiotic Use (which could kill the normal, beneficial bacteria present in the intestines)
- Lactose Intolerance
- Major Colon Diseases (such as diverticular disease)
- Allergies
- Parasites
- Disease-Causing Bacteria

## Control Symptoms Through Proper Diet

Here are some general guidelines that will help you control IBS symptoms:

1. Avoid all coffee, tea, alcohol, and tobacco.
2. Try a vegetarian diet! For best results, give special emphasis to raw fruits and vegetables and foods that are high in fiber, low in fat, and low in protein.
3. Eat whole-grain cereal. Rice bran and oat bran are excellent sources of fiber. If you take raw millers bran, drink plenty of liquids. If you are constipated, bran will not irritate (laxatives may), and bran can be mixed with other foods or with juice.
4. If you have a sensitivity to wheat, eat whole-grain rye bread, and for fiber, substitute corn bran or buckwheat groats (kasha).
5. Include other excellent sources of fiber in your diet such as cabbage, dried fruit, apples, prunes, carrots, peas, spinach, bananas, pears, beets, corn, and dried beans.
6. Increase your intake of sprouted seeds, such as alfalfa, mungbean, and sunflower.
7. Avoid milk and milk products. Reason: Many people who have IBS are sensitive to milk sugar; that is, they have lactose intolerance.

## Specific Remedies

Here are some specific remedies to help you cope with IBS:

*For Constipation:* For seven to ten days, fast on the juices listed under Juice Therapy on page 115.

*For Diarrhea—The Acute Phase:* During the acute phase of diarrhea: Increase your fluid intake. Use electrolyte and trace-mineral formulas to prevent the depletion of minerals in your system. Take acidophilus (Megadophilus brand) to stabilize your healthy intestinal bacteria. Acidophilus is especially helpful if the diarrhea is caused by antibiotics. For three or four days avoid all food except for some grated apple with a pinch of cinnamon.

*As Conditions Improve*: As the diarrhea eases, add cultured-milk products such as yogurt, kefir, and buttermilk, as well as bananas, ripe papaya, blueberries, and whole grains. Bananas and raw millers bran are very effective in cases of chronic diarrhea.

Follow this classic folk remedy for good results: Eat one to four tablespoons of scraped apple every hour. Also, take in plenty of fluids and essential minerals and three tablespoons of unsweetened carob powder daily.

Remember that lactose may trigger your symptoms, so avoid all milk products.

*For Bloating and Flatulence:* Avoid foods that might produce gas: for example, onions, beans, lentils, wheat germ, celery, carrots, and brussels sprouts.

Keep a diary of what you eat each day. Your written notes may help you find out whether any specific foods trigger IBS symptoms.

## Juice Therapy

A number of healing juices are effective for IBS symptoms:

| | | |
|---|---|---|
| Spinach | Cucumber | Beet |
| Watercress | Celery | Tomato |
| Carrot | Cabbage | |

In addition, here are some specific juice therapies for constipation and diarrhea:

*For Constipation:* Add 1 tablespoon of raw millers bran to a combination of apple, blueberry, and lemon juices.

*For Diarrhea:* Do not use juices in the acute phase of diarrhea. Take juices only as healing begins to take place. Then drink a combination of carrot, alfalfa, sprout, and beet juice to which you've added a trace-mineral supplement.

## Helpful Herbs

Herbs that are generally helpful in IBS conditions are:

| | |
|---|---|
| Psyllium seed husks | Buckhorn bark |
| Alfalfa tablets | Raspberry leaves |
| Aloe vera | Slippery elm bark gruel |
| Cascara sagrada | Peppermint tea |
| Unsweetened carob powder | Licorice |

In addition, here are some specific remedies:

*For Diarrhea:* Take unsweetened carob powder. It has a high pectin content and therefore acts as an excellent binder for loose bowels. In addition, chew raw garlic, make a witch hazel tea, or try raspberry leaves.

Another remedy is to take a combination of kaolin and apple pectin—for example, Kaopectate.

*For Constipation:* Take bentonite, a type of volcanic ash, combined with psyllium seed husks. The combination is very effective for constipation.

## Aroma Therapy

For colonic spasms, use peppermint oil. For diarrhea, add 15 drops of essence of peppermint oil to a cup of hot water, and take this every three hours.

## Acupressure and Massage

Abdominal rocking, abdominal kneading, and massage will help reduce the discomfort caused by gas trapped in the intestine.

## Exercise

Race walking, stretching, and swimming regularly are especially effective in treating IBS. Also, try yoga breathing exercises.

## Hydrotherapy

Several hydrotherapy techniques will help relieve the symptoms of IBS:

*For Abdominal Gas:* Place a wet heating pad over the abdomen to reduce gas pains.

*For Constipation:* Take a high-pressure cold-water shower. Spray the shower on the back of your body in the following sequence:

Begin at your right heel. Then move the spray to:

1. The top of the buttocks.
2. The left heel.
3. The top of the buttocks.
4. The right buttock.
5. The right shoulder.
6. The right buttock again.
7. The left buttock.
8. The left shoulder.
9. The left heel.

Then spray the shower on the front of your body in the following sequence: Begin at your right foot. Then move the spray to:

1. The top of the right hip bone.
2. The left foot.
3. The top of the left hip bone.
4. The right shoulder.
5. The right hip bone again.
6. The left hip bone again.
7. The left shoulder.
8. The left foot.

For related remedies, see pages 217 and 218 of the Appendix.

## Emotions and IBS

People who suffer from IBS often suffer from depression too. Depression can be the result of food sensitivity. Therefore, it certainly is worthwhile to undergo some food-sensitivity tests or seek counseling and psychotherapy.

## Homeopathy

Try whichever of these homeopathic approaches is appropriate to your symptoms:

*For an Addiction to Laxatives:* Take one dose of nux vomica before you go to bed.

*For Constipation:* If you have a rectal fissure and find it painful to pass stool, take sulfur to get back to normal.

*For Difficulty Passing Stool:* If your stool is soft and sticky and you must use lots of toilet paper, try alumina.

*For Large, Hard, Dry Stools:* Take bryonia.

*For Diarrhea Caused by Fear or Stress:* Take gelsemium.

*For Watery, Yellow Stools:* Take podophyllum for watery, yellow stools that squirt out after meals or early in the morning.

*For Changing Diarrhea:* If the form of diarrhea is sometimes watery, sometimes slimy, and the stool is filled with undigested food, take sulfur.

## Tissue Salts

For chronic constipation, alternate taking sodium phosphate and sodium sulfate.
   For diarrhea, try whichever of the following is most appropriate:

- For diarrhea caused by parasites or worms, take sodium phosphate.
- For general diarrhea in children, try phosphate of iron.
- For diarrhea caused by a poor diet of rich and fatty foods (as indicated by a coated tongue), take potassium chloride.
- For diarrhea caused by emotional upset, take potassium phosphate.
- For diarrhea alternating with constipation, take phosphate of iron and calcium phosphate.

## Tips to Remember

If you suffer from IBS, you might benefit from these miscellaneous notes:

- You can eliminate or drastically reduce abdominal gas by eating slowly and by avoiding drinking carbonated beverages, chewing gum, and sucking candy.
- If you are constipated, try this technique: Place a small footstool in front of your toilet seat. When you sit on the toilet bowl, rest your feet on the footstool and lean your body forward. Take long, deep breaths to facilitate the bowel movement.
- Try charcoal tablets for relieving diarrhea.

## David C. Cures Constipation With Natural Healing

For more than 20 years, David C. suffered from constipation. He had no more than three movements a week, and these few movements were very painful.
   One day he decided to consult a nutritionist, who reviewed David's dietary habits, of course, and discovered that David suffered from irritated bowel syndrome.
   As a result of a complete study, the nutritionist told David to:

- Eliminate all refined carbohydrates, coffee, tea, and alcohol from his diet.
- Have a breakfast of: (1) one tablespoon of raw millers bran added to a combination of carrot, celery, and beet juice; and (2) four or five dried figs that had been soaked in distilled water overnight.
- Eat macrobiotic-style meals: Combine beans and whole grains such as brown rice, pasta, millet, or buckwheat. Include a sea vegetable of some type, for example, hiziki or wakamae. Add 2 tablespoons of olive oil to each meal.
- Eat one meal of a fruit that is in season.
- Eat one meal of a salad and steamed vegetables.
- Supplement each meal with 3 alfalfa tablets and a glass of licorice root tea during the day.
- Do nonstop abdominal-strenghtening exercises every day, beginning with two minutes and adding one minute every week until he reached ten minutes of nonstop exercise a day. Walk or swim laps for at least 30 minutes each day. Stretch for 10 minutes before each workout.

• Have a professional Swedish massage twice a week. With special attention to his abdominal muscles, his colon will become less spastic.

What were the results of David's new regimen? In the beginning, David experienced even more flatulence than usual, as the herbs and fiber increased the movement of gas out of his intestinal tract. But gradually, David began having three or four full bowel movements each day! After a month on the new program, he replaced figs with a whole-grain cereal and soy milk at breakfast, and he lowered the number of alfalfa tablets each morning to *one*.

Through natural healing techniques, David C. was able to overcome his long-established constipation problems. As long as he stays on this healthy program, he will continue to have normal, full bowel movements.

# 26

# Jet Lag

The frequency with which people now fly anywhere in the world for business or pleasure makes jet lag a common ailment among many, many people each day. Of course, for the person who travels often, jet lag is more than a minor nuisance.

Basically, jet lag is the result of the body's inability to readjust its internal time clock to new time zones. Essentially, our body rhythms are thrown off by the time changes. But despite its name, jet lag is not restricted to fliers and travelers. It affects shift workers—people who must change their working hours periodically. They, too, can suffer the same effects.

## Avoiding Jet Lag with the Argonne Anti-Jet Lag Diet

Perhaps the most effective method for avoiding jet lag is the Argonne Anti-Jet Lag Diet, which was developed by Dr. Charles F. Ehret of the Argonne National Laboratory's Division of Biological and Medical Research. With certain modifications, the dietary recommendations about to be discussed are based on this well-known diet. [Charles F. Ehret and Lynn Waller Scanlon, *Overcoming Jet Lag*, New York, Berkeley Books, 1983.]

To avoid the effects of jet lag, follow these steps:

1. Determine what breakfast time will be when you arrive at your destination.

2. On home time, beginning three days before you depart, *feast-fast-feast-fast*, as explained here:

*Day 1:* On Day #1, feast. Eat a hearty high-protein breakfast and a high-carbohydrate dinner. But be sure to drink no coffee!

*Day 2:* Fast on light meals—salads, light soups, fruits, and juices.

*Day 3:* Feast again, as on Day #1.

*Day 4:* Fast! This is departure day. Avoid any caffeinated beverages. If you are traveling west, you may fast for only half the day. (If you insist on having caffeinated beverages, drink them only in the morning when traveling west, or between 6 and 11 p.m. when traveling east.)

3. When you reach your destination, break your final fast at breakfast time. In the meantime, do not drink any alcohol on the plane. If the flight is long enough, sleep until the normal breakfast time at your destination—but no later.

4. When you wake up, feast on a high-protein breakfast. Stay awake and stay active! Continue your day's meals according to the meal times at your destination.

*Feasting at Breakfast and Lunch.* Use high-protein foods to stimulate your body's active cycle. Suitable foods include unsweetened yogurt, buttermilk, a cheese sandwich on whole-grain bread (avoid pasteurized process cheese foods and American cheese), high-protein cereal with soy milk or skim milk, green beans and legumes, tofu, tempeh, and a high-protein health shake.

*Feasting at Supper.* To stimulate sleep, eat high-complex carbohydrates, for example: whole-grain pasta, cereal, breads, potatoes, squash (or other starchy vegetables), fruit, desserts sweetened with fruit juice or barley malt, and syrup (these desserts are available in natural food stores).

Avoid protein foods.

*Fasting Days.* Fasting days help the liver to store carbohydrates and prepare the body's clock for resetting. Suitable foods include: fruit, light vegetable broths and soups (dry, packaged mixes made from high-quality ingredients are available in most natural food stores), green and mixed vegetable salads, and unbuttered whole-grain toast.

Keep calories and carbohydrates to a minimum.

## Tryptophane and Jet Lag

The use of tryptophane has been found to greatly reduce nausea during your flight. Take 500 milligrams several hours before the flight and another 500 milligrams during the flight.

## Ginger and Nausea

Use ginger tea or take ginger herbal capsules to reduce nausea during your flight.

## Tips to Remember

Bright sunlight sends a strong environmental message that helps your body rhythms to readjust. Therefore, take a brisk walk soon after your arrival.

## For More Information

If you'd like to learn more about the Argonne Anti-Jet Lag Diet, you may wish to read *Overcoming Jet Lag* (see page 119), or you may contact:

Office of Public Affairs
Argonne National Laboratory
9700 South Cass Avenue
Argonne, IL 60439

# 27

# Liver Problems

The liver is the largest organ in the body. Far more important than its size, the liver performs more functions than any other organ.

The liver serves as the body's primary organ for the metabolism of carbohydrates, fats, and proteins. In addition, the liver performs the primary cleaning functions of the body, a job that increases the chances of the liver's being damaged by drugs and alcohol.

## Common Liver Disorders

*Cirrhosis.* This chronic disease may result from viral hepatitis, malnutrition, alcoholism, chronic inflammation of certain ducts in the liver, or obstruction of those ducts. As a result of cirrhosis, liver cells degenerate and scar.

*Hepatitis.* An inflammation of the liver, hepatitis can cause flu-like symptoms: Yellowing of the white areas of the eyes, brown urine, chills, fever, nausea, diarrhea, swollen lymph glands, tenderness in the stomach area between the ribs, and acute discomfort below the rib cage on the right side of the body.

Actually, there are three different varieties of hepatitis:

1. *Infectious Hepatitis.* Also called "Type A," infectious hepatitis may exhibit no symptoms, or it may exhibit all hepatitis symptoms.

2. *Serum hepatitis.* This is Type B hepatitis, which is generally transmitted by unsanitary hypodermic needles.

3. *Toxic Hepatitis.* As its name implies, this variety of hepatitis is caused by toxic agents, such as chemicals and drugs.

*Gilbert's Disease.* A liver dysfunction characterized by intermittent low-grade jaundice.

*Fatty Liver.* Fatty liver is generally caused by protein deficiency (common in alcoholics) or by uncontrolled diabetes.

*Acute Yellow Atrophy.* In this disease, the liver cells suddenly die, and the liver ceases to function. The causes are alcohol abuse and/or malnutrition, but acute yellow atrophy may possibly also be caused by pregnancy, yellow fever, and serum hepatitis.

## Good Nutrition: The Key to Liver Therapy

To cleanse the liver and begin a nutritional program for keeping the liver clean and healthy, follow these suggestions:

• Fast on juices for seven to ten days using the recommendations listed under Juice Therapy on page 124.

• Every morning, prepare this "liver flush" tea, which will cleanse the liver, the digestive tract, and the intestines:

> 1 teaspoon olive oil
> ½ teaspoon fresh ginger
> 1 teaspoon fenugreek
> The juice of 1 whole lemon
> A pinch of capsicum

Take 1 cup boiling distilled water; let the water cool for one or two minutes before adding the above ingredients. Add the olive oil *last*, just before you are ready to drink the tea.

Strain the mixture and drink the liquid. If you prefer, you may liquefy the ingredients in a blender and then drink the tea. [This is a modified version of the "liver flush" developed by Dr. Randolph Stone, the developer of the Polarity Therapy healing system.]

• Eat small meals frequently rather than few large meals.

• Eliminate all fats and oils from your diet for several weeks.

• After the juice fast, follow a lactovegetarian diet using only organically grown foods.

• Eat plenty of high-quality protein, which is essential for healing the liver. The best choices are:

Goat's milk

Brewer's yeast

Raw-milk cottage cheese

Sprouted seeds and grains

Raw and unsalted nuts and seeds

Nut and seed butters (especially almond butter)

• Avoid canned, frozen, or otherwise processed foods.

• Avoid fats and oils for two to three weeks, as well as fried, fatty, and oily foods. If you must use any oil, use only virgin light olive oil.

• Avoid sugar, salt, and any strong spices, including black and white pepper, mustard, and clove.

- Chew all your foods well.
- Include these foods in your diet: apples, asparagus, beets, celery, endive, artichoke, cucumber, garlic, and lemon. Apples, asparagus, and celery are old folk remedies for stimulating a sluggish liver.

## Specific Therapies for Liver Diseases

*For general liver problems:*

- Fast for 3 to 7 days on carrots and apples. Three times a day, add 20 drops of Oregon grape root to the carrots or apples.
- Place castor oil packs over the liver before bedtime for four evenings.

*For Jaundice:* Follow a strict macrobiotic diet. Eat grains, beans, sea vegetables, tofu, and so on. Use plenty of daikon radish and mugwort tea every day.

*For Cirrhosis:* A high-protein diet (75 to 100 grams a day) is a must for anyone suffering from cirrhosis because protein regenerates liver cells. Also, to increase the glycogen stored by the body, follow a program high in calories (300 to 400 calories a day) and high in complex carbohydrates. The glycogen ensures that the protein will be used to regenerate liver cells rather than used for energy. In addition, the glycogen helps compensate for the weight loss that generally results from fever in cirrhosis cases.

## Amino Acid Therapy

Amino acids serve specific purposes in helping the liver:

- Aspartic acid serves a protective function for the liver.
- Carnitine may reverse alcohol-induced liver damage.
- Methionine has a lipotropic function: it prevents deposits and cohesion of fats in the liver. Always take vitamin $B_6$ whenever you take methionine.
- Arginine detoxifies ammonia and is therefore useful in treating cirrhosis.

## Supplements Are Mandatory

The liver is involved in making certain vitamins available to the body in their active form. Therefore, an unhealthy liver can cause many nutritional complications. As you can see, then, supplementation plays an especially important role both in helping the liver to recuperate from disease and in maintaining its normal healthy state.

Some nutrients that are effective in a health-building program for the liver are:

*Whey.* For general liver problems, add one teaspoon of whey to 8 ounces of water.

*Niacin.* Although niacin is necessary for healthy liver function, mega doses of niacin or niacinamide can cause liver dysfunction and liver damage. Do not use mega doses unless you are under the care of a competent health professional.

*Vitamin A:* High doses (that is, over 50,000 iu) of vitamin A can cause a toxic reaction in the liver. Unless you are under the care of a competent health professional, do not take high doses of vitamin A.

For specific liver conditions, follow these recommendations:

*For Hepatitis:* In doses from 20 to 50 grams daily, vitamin C (as sodium ascorbate) can help you recover from this viral infection. Such large doses should be administered intravenously three or four times a day (only by a physician, of course). Because large doses of vitamin C remove calcium and other minerals from the body, your physician should add calcium to the IV solution. According to Dr. Jonathan Wright, the extra calcium will help avoid abnormal muscle contractions. [Jonathan V. Wright, *Dr. Wright's Book of Nutritional Therapy*, Emmaus, Pennsylvania, Rodale Press, 1979, p. 262.]

*For Fatty Liver:* The liver regulates cholesterol levels in the body with the help of certain nutrients: vitamin $B_{12}$, lecithin, choline, biotin, and calcium pangamate.

Nutritional deficiencies, on the other hand, can contribute to fatty liver—specifically, deficiencies in:

| | | |
|---|---|---|
| Chromium | Vitamin $B_6$ | Vanadium |
| Manganese | Niacin | Vitamin C |
| Selenium | Magnesium | Vitamin E |
| Zinc | Potassium | Folic acid |

## Juice Therapy

For a healthy liver, try these juice therapy recommendations:

• Drink Juice Therapy Formula #18 or #25 (twice daily).

• Squeeze ten lemons in two quarts of water and drink a glass of the mixture every two hours. Sweeten with honey or maple syrup if you wish.

• For an enlarged liver, drink papaya juice.

• Grape juice is also a very good healing juice for the liver.

• Drink a combination of carrot, beet, and dandelion juices.

• To promote bile activity, add lemon juice to water and drink this mixture in the morning.

## Herbal Remedies for a Healthy Liver

For some specific herbal remedies, consider the following recommendations:

• Use the "liver flush" tea described on page 122.

• Drink centaury tea before a meal. This bitter tonic will stimulate the liver and increase bile action.

• For hepatitis, try this remedy: Boil one teaspoon of dandelion roots in eight ounces of distilled water for about ten minutes. Strain the roots, and allow the mixture to cool. Drink six to eight ounces each day for five to six weeks.

• Combine milk thistle, artichoke, and curcuma—or if you prefer, buy the commercial preparation, Silymarin Complex (see "For More Information").

• Make a poultice of peppermint tea with a pinch of cinnamon, and apply the poultice over the liver.

## Aroma Therapy

For general liver disorders, try these essences: lemon, rosemary, thyme, peppermint, or sage.

## Acupressure and Massage

Try full-body muscle rock. Also, follow the instructions for Circular Rhythmic Pressure in the chart in the Appendix.

## Homeopathy

To a glass of distilled water, add 1 teaspoon of white or yellow clay and several drops of Lachesis 12X or 10X. [From A. Vogel, *Swiss Nature Doctor*, Switzerland, A. Vogel, 19--, p. 213.]

## Tissue Salts

For indigestion due to a sluggish liver, take calcium phosphate, potassium phosphate, and sodium chloride.

For general liver disorders and biliousness, take sodium sulfate 6X.

## Hydrotherapy

Apply continuous warm castor oil packs over the liver area. Also, apply hot ginger or taro potato compresses over the liver.

Follow this tip from *Herbal Medicine: The Natural Way to Get Well and Stay Well*:

"Burdock leaf packs are useful on the inflamed liver area. Alternate them with castor oil packs or peppermint and cinnamon packs." [Dian Dincin Buchman, *Herbal Medicine: The Natural Way to Get Well and Stay Well*, N.Y., Gramercy Publishing Co., 1979, p. 163.]

## For More Information

The Silymarin Complex mentioned earlier is available from:

Enzymatic Therapy, Inc.
P.O. Box 1508
Green Bay, WI 54305
414-437-1061

# 28

# Male Sexual and Reproductive Problems

Many of the sexual and reproductive problems that are specific to men may be helped by natural healing methods. Two of the most common male sexual and reproductive problems are impotence and infertility, which are discussed further:

## Impotence

Impotence is the inability to get or maintain an erection well enough for complete intercourse. The causes of impotence may be emotional, or the causes may be physical. Impotence is not a "normal" result of aging, as many people incorrectly believe.

Among the factors that can lead to impotence are:

- Arteriosclerosis
- Hypertension
- Diabetes
- Brain or spinal cord injuries
- Surgical removal of the prostate gland, bladder, or rectum
- Radiation treatment for cancer

- Tobacco, drug, and alcohol use
- Certain medications (especially medications used to treat high blood pressure and depression)

In many instances, impotence can be cured. The first step is to identify the *cause* of the problem.

## Infertility

Infertility is the inability of a couple to achieve pregnancy despite regular sexual activity (without contraceptives) for a period of one year or more.

Infertility in the male may be caused by:

- *A low sperm count*, which can result from a number of causes, such as environmental exposure to chemicals; excessive heat in the workplace; excessive use of alcohol, tobacco, or caffeine; or use of certain prescription drugs (note that the side effects of all drugs are enclosed in drug packages.)
- *Prostate gland enlargement*, which is known as "benign prostatic hypertrophy" or just BPH. BPH generally interferes with intercourse and urination. Its symptoms may include pain or burning during urination; hesitation or difficulty in urinating; feelings of pressure and fullness in the bladder and in the anal area; and dribbling at the end of urination or afterward.

BPH is usually accompanied by some degree of inflammation.

- *Prostatitis*, which is an inflammation of the prostate gland. In young men, prostatitis is usually caused by a bacterial infection. The symptoms of prostatitis include fever, pain between the scrotum and the rectum, blood or pus in the urine, and frequent urination accompanied by a burning sensation.
- *Spermagglutination*, a disorder that causes sperm cells to stick together and, therefore, restricts the mobility of sperm cells.

## The General Role of Nutrition

A number of nutrients can be very beneficial in the conditions previously discussed.

***Zinc and EFAs.*** Zinc is essential for healthy sexual functioning. This trace mineral helps in the formation of active sperm in *all* mammals and in the production and function of several sex hormones.

A severe zinc deficiency may result in smaller sex organs and in male sterility. A deficiency of essential fatty acids (EFAs) may contribute to prostate gland enlargement.

Because pumpkin seeds are good sources of both zinc and EFAs, they are considered of great value in prostate problems.

***Selenium.*** Based on preliminary studies, many nutritionists believe that selenium is vital for normal reproduction.

***Vitamin A.*** A deficiency of vitamin A can cause degeneration and loss of sperm cells.

***Vitamin C.*** In a 1979 study, vitamin C increased sperm count by 54 percent.

*Vitamin E.* Vitamin E is important in the production of certain hormones that trigger the male sex drive.

## The Specific Role of Nutrition

In addition to the general roles discussed above, nutritional remedies can help in specific male sexual and reproductive disorders.

*Prostate Gland Enlargement (or BPH).* If you suffer from an enlarged prostate, cut down on your use of dairy products, meats, and all other foods that are high in cholesterol. Reason: Studies show that when cholesterol levels are reduced, enlarged prostates, too, are reduced.

Also, avoid tobacco and certain spices. BPH symptoms clear up or improve when use of these "urothelial irritants," as they are called, are discontinued.

*Prostatitis.* Increase your intake of fluids if you have prostatitis. Also, if you have fever, increase your intake of protein and calories. Avoid alcohol, caffeine, and spicy foods. Eat sunflower seeds or sesame seed oil, both of which contain EFAS. EFA deficiency may contribute to prostate problems.

## Amino Acid Therapy

A number of amino acids can be very helpful in cases of sexual and reproductive problems:

*Arginine.* This amino acid can increase sperm count and sperm motility.

*GABA (Gamma-Aminobutryic Acid).* GABA may help reduce an enlarged prostate gland by suppressing prolactia, which is released by the pituitary gland.

*Histadine.* Histadine releases histamines from body stores. Histamines are necessary for sexual arousal.

*Phenylalanine.* Recent studies show that phenylalanine can affect emotional factors that, in turn, may limit sexual ability.

*Glutamic Acid, Alanine, and Glycine (Aminoacetic Acid).* Studies show that a combination of these three amino acids can successfully reduce the symptoms of prostate gland enlargement (BPH). This mixture is available under the brand name Prostex Amino Acid Formula. (See "For More Information" on page 130 for a source of Prostex.)

## Bee Pollen—A Valuable Supplement

Many natural healers consider bee pollen especially important in maintaining sexual health. Bee pollen contains a natural substance that works as a specific nutrient for the sex glands. Further, studies at a university in Yugoslavia showed that men who used bee pollen had increased self-confidence and sexual performance.

Another valuable supplement, *octacosanol*, increases fertility and sperm production.

In addition to bee pollen and octacosanol, other supplements are effective in specific male conditions, for example:

*For Prostate Problems:* The supplements that are helpful in prostate conditions are: vitamin E, EFAs, zinc, vitamin A, and calcium.

These nutrients—especially zinc—produced great relief from prostate symptoms when taken over a 6- to 8-month period.

*For Spermagglutination:* In 1979 lab tests, results showed that a preparation containing vitamin C, calcium, magnesium, and manganese reversed spermagglutination conditions and raised sperm counts.

## Juice Therapy

Try Juice Therapy Formula #6 (see the Appendix). Also, drink these two juice combinations: (1) Mix carrot and spinach juices; and (2) Mix carrot, asparagus, and lettuce juices.

## Effective Herbs

Among the herbs that are considered effective in male sexual and reproductive conditions are:

| | |
|---|---|
| Echinacea | Sarsaparilla |
| Saw palmetto | Yohimbe |
| Juniper berry | Marsh mallow |
| Damiana | Capsicum |
| Ginger root | Uva ursi |
| Horsetail grass | Parsley root |
| Hydrangea root | Ginseng |
| Prickly ash bark | Birch leaf |

## Aroma Therapy

Ylang-ylang oil is considered a mild nerve stimulant and aphrodisiac. Essences used for specific conditions are:

*For Impotence:* Cinnamon, clover, peppermint, pine, ginger, juniper, onion, thyme, rosemary, sandalwood, and savory.

*For Prostate Gland Enlargement (BPH):* Essence of onion and essence of thuja.

*For Prostatitis:* Essence of pine.

## Acupressure and Massage

Try deep rhythmic pressure (see chart in the Appendix) and nerve strokes.

## Exercise

Try tai chi and yoga breathing exercises.

In addition, "Healing Tao" is recommended by many natural healers for health problems in general and sexual problems in particular. Healing Tao is a Chinese system of body/mind/spirit disciplines that tries to balance sexual energy. See "For More Information" on page 130 for the address of the Healing Tao Center.

## Hydrotherapy

In acute conditions, try hot chamomile sitz baths for relief from symptoms.

## Homeopathy

Use saw palmetto for prostate enlargement and for difficulty in urination. In addition, you may try chimaphila or sulfur for prostate enlargement.

## Tissue Salts

The tissue salts that are most effective in prostatitis (painful urination) are phosphate of iron, calcium fluoride, and silicic oxide.

## Tips to Remember

• Early puberty can be brought on by an excessive intake of sugar, according to *Prevention Magazine* (October 1975, pp. 178-184).

• Heavy alcohol use can cause the body to lose zinc and thus contribute to prostate gland enlargement.

• In prostatitis conditions, try to avoid exposure to very cold weather.

• For general sexual health, avoid deliberately prolonging ejaculation. Suppressing ejaculation can contribute to functional or structural damage.

• To improve semen quality, men can wear scrotal pouches, which allow evaporative cooling of the testes, according to *The Lancet* (April 26, 1980).

## For More Information

To find out more about Healing Tao (discussed on page 129), contact:

Healing Tao Center
P.O. Box 1194
Huntington, NY 11743
(516) 549-9452

The Prostex Amino Acid Formula is available from:

Advance Laboratories, Inc.
120 Elm Street
Watertown, MA 02172
(617) 926-0801

A good source of general information is the Sex Information and Education Council of the U.S. (SIECUS):

SIECUS
84 Fifth Avenue (Suite 407)
New York, NY 10011

# 29

# Memory Loss

Forgetting things is perfectly normal, that is, to a certain degree. When we say "memory loss," we are referring to abnormal, perhaps preventable forgetfulness; the kind of condition that might be improved through good nutrition.

## Facts Concerning Memory

Recent studies show that, contrary to long-held beliefs, gradual memory loss over time is not "normal." True, certain types of memory may diminish with age, but remembering names and faces, for example, does not diminish with age. Likewise, "prospective memory," the ability to remember to do a task at a certain time, does not diminish with age. [Daniel Goleman, "Forgetfulness Is Seen Causing More Worry Than It Should," *New York Times*, July 1, 1986, p. C9.]

## Life Style Affects Memory

Interestingly, your life style can contribute to forgetfulness:

* People who claim to have "internal alarms" and people who trust their memory instead of writing themselves notes tend to complain more about missing appointments.

* Did you ever look for something in a certain place, continue looking elsewhere, and then find the misplaced object in a spot you had already searched? The cause may be a perceptual problem, rather than memory loss, which is often mistakenly blamed.

* Forgetting may be a convenient way to overlook obligations or avoid unpleasant feelings.

## Good Nutrition Can Help

Acetylcholine, a chemical found in the brain, is responsible for transmitting messages from one brain cell to another. Acetylcholine is a very important factor in memory retention, and low levels of this essential substance can affect memory.

Consider these recommendations:

• Use soybeans as a source of phosphatidyl choline, the form of choline that helps improve memory and mental function in general.

• Avoid using aluminum cookware. Although this topic is admittedly controversial, many natural healers have long believed that aluminum from cookware can enter the body and negatively affect normal brain function.

## Supplements Are Effective

Certain nutrients can be beneficial in helping to prevent memory loss and retain normal brain function:

• *Vitamin $B_{12}$* stimulates the production of RNA (ribonucleic acid), which is necessary for memory and learning.

• *Choline* may improve memory in adults over college age. In one study, college students who were given choline were better able to recall lengthy word sequences.

• *Pantothenic acid*, a B vitamin, may improve memory by helping to transform choline and phosphatidyl choline into acetylcholine.

• *Iron* increases the body's use of oxygen, which is essential for effective brain function, of course. Even normal levels of iron can affect memory and alertness if these normal levels are low.

• *Vitamin $B_1$* deficiency (common in alcoholics) can affect short-term memory.

## Effective Herbs

Also be sure to include the following herbs in your diet:

| | |
|---|---|
| Gotu kola capsules (250 mg.) | Prickly ash bark |
| Fo ti capsules (125 mg.) | Hawthorn berries |
| Periwinkle | Rosemary leaves |
| Capsicum | Ginseng |

## Aroma Therapy

Try the following essences: rosemary, coriander, and clove.

## Exercise

Studies show that a combination of (1) a high-fiber diet and (2) daily walks improved intellectual efficiency. In general, people who exercise have better memories than people who lead sedentary lives.

# 30

# Menopause

Menopause, the cessation of menses, is a natural condition. It occurs gradually over a period of time; in most cases, anywhere from a few months to 5 years. In exceptional cases, menopause may last up to 10 years.

## Estrogen Production Slows Down

During menopause, a woman's body slows down its estrogen production, which in turn slows down both the duration of menstruation and the amount of the menstrual flow. But until the change is complete and menses ceases, the body's hormonal balance is uneven and irregular. As a result, menstruation is erratic: one month, menstrual flow may be light; the next month, heavy. Even if menstruation ceases altogether for several months, it may begin again.

Generally, women between age 45 and age 53 who have not menstruated in one year or more have probably completed menopause.

## Hot Flashes and Other Symptoms

Various symptoms may accompany menopause, including:

- Hot flashes, accompanied by a tingling sensation, chills, sweating, and headaches
- Fatigue
- Frequent urination
- Palpitations
- Slightly increased blood pressure
- Giddiness
- Slight water retention

- Nausea
- Loss of appetite
- Insomnia
- Mood swings
- Anxiety

Except for hot flashes, these symptoms may really be an emotional response to the onset of menopause, or they may be caused by other factors unrelated to menopause—for example, problems concerning a woman's career, her family and friends, her health, or other business and personal concerns.

Hot flashes were once considered an emotional reaction, but recent research has shown that *hot flashes* are well named. The temperature of a woman's skin *can* actually increase during a "hot flash." In addition to feeling this temperature change, a woman may also feel tingling, chills, and cold sweats. But the cause of hot flashes is not yet known. Perhaps stress may be a contributing factor.

## Good Diet Can Help

To help offset some of the symptoms of menopause, follow these recommendations:

- Avoid alcohol, coffee, and other stimulants.
- Avoid taking any depressant agents.
- Follow a lactovegetarian diet, which eliminates meat, fish, eggs and poultry, but allows the use of milk products.

## Supplements Can Help

Three supplements that are especially helpful in connection with menopause are L-Tryptophan, vitamin E, and vitamin C.

*L-Tryptophan* is very helpful in cases of postmenopausal depression, the depression that women sometimes experience after menopause. *Vitamin E* can be very effective in reducing—and even eliminating—hot flashes associated with menopause, especially when vitamin E is taken together with vitamin C. Take 2,000-3,000 iu for hot flashes; otherwise, take only 800 iu daily. NOTE: Do not take a high dose if you have high blood pressure.

*Vitamin C* when taken together with bioflavonoids can also reduce hot flashes. Take 2,000-3,000 mg. daily.

## Juice Therapy

Use Juice Therapy Formulas #2 and #6, which are described in the Appendix.

Also, try drinking a glass of ice water at the first sign of symptoms.

## Herbal Remedies

Herbs that are effective during menopause include:

| | | |
|---|---|---|
| Lobelia | Black Cohosh root | Shepherd's purse |
| Meadowsweet | Red raspberry leaves | Unicorn root |
| Ginger root | Cayenne pepper | Licorice root |
| Goldenseal root | Elder flowers | Marsh mallow root |

Here is a special formula for menopausal symptoms recommended by Humbart Santillo in *Natural Healing With Herbs* [Hohm Press, 1984, p. 332]:

Combine *1 part each* of the following herbs in powdered form:

| | |
|---|---|
| Ginger root | Squaw vine |
| Black haw | Licorice root |
| Helonias root | Dong quai |
| Siberian ginseng | |

Make capsules from the mixed powder using #00 gelatin capsules. Take 2 capsules twice a day with meals or when symptoms occur. (As an alternative to capsules, you may take the powder in rice paper.)

## Acupressure and Massage

Kneading on the abdomen and the back of the legs and arms is also helpful for menopausal symptoms. In addition, try circular rhythmic pressure. See the chart on page *000*.

Dry brushing also helps to reduce menopausal symptoms. Every day, dry brush your entire body with a loofah or a terry cloth towel.

## Hydrotherapy

Try hot and cold packs over the upper spine. Also, try alternating hot and cold showers.

## Homeopathy

Here are some useful homeopathic remedies:

- For hot flashes and other symptoms of menopause: Sanguinaria or sepia.
- For hot flashes, headaches, and climate changes: Lachesis.
- For irritability: Salix nig.

## Aroma Therapy

Use these essences for menopausal symptoms: chamomile, cypress, and sage.

## Exercise

Regular aerobic exercises and yoga are highly recommended during menopause and afterward.

## Tips to Remember

- Weight may effect the onset of menopause. In a Belgian study, women who weighed more than 132 pounds went through menopause later.
- Women who smoke experience menopause earlier, according to a report in *The Lancet* [June 25, 1977].

# 31

# Musculoskeletal Problems

As the name clearly tells, *musculoskeletal* describes the complex system of muscles and bones that make up your body. Of all the causes that can be responsible for various musculoskeletal problems, one clearly stands out above all the rest: *poor posture*.

## The Effects of Poor Posture

Many authorities agree that poor posture may actually contribute to certain organic diseases. Poor posture may constrict lung function. When your shoulders are rounded, your breathing is inhibited because your lungs cannot expand properly. As a result, you can neither inhale as much oxygen nor exhale as much carbon dioxide! Such poor breathing can reduce your energy levels and create a toxic condition in your body.

What causes us to stand or sit improperly? Among the primary causes of poor posture are:

* Weakened muscles, especially (1) the muscles that support the spine and (2) the abdominal and chest muscles that support the front of the body and hold the body upright.

* Emotional trauma.

* Improper balance and alignment of the feet.

## Practice Good Posture Every Day

To maintain good posture, practice these few techniques *every day*:

*When Sitting:* Use a straight-back, L-shape chair whenever possible, and always push your buttocks as far back into the chair as possible!

*When Standing and Walking:* Be aware of your shoulders. Do not tighten up or push your shoulders forward. You should be able to move your arms about freely. Further, your chest should feel open and unconstricted.

*When Sleeping:* For proper sleeping posture, see the section on "Sleep Disorders."

## Orthotic Devices Can Help

Your feet are the structural foundation for all the weight-bearing joints in your body. When you stand or walk, you body weight should be supported properly by your knees, hips, sacroiliac, and spinal joints. Any imbalance in bearing your body weight will cause a musculoskeletal disorder.

An *orthotic* is a special device used to correct any postural imbalance that arises as a result of abnormal foot function. Specifically, an orthotic reduces musculoskeletal stress and strain caused by the imbalance. Many people, especially athletes, have reported feeling dramatic relief from musculoskeletal conditions as a result of wearing an orthotic device.

Of course, the orthotic must be properly fitted by a orthopedist, podiatrist, chiropractor or a sports medicine doctor, who will carefully and precisely measure your feet and make molds in the process of creating the device.

## Common Musculoskeletal Disorders

Among the most common musculoskeletal disorders are these:

*Back Pain.* There are many different types of back pain. Even in those back conditions that are caused by abnormalities or structural damage, however, tension plays a major role. As a result of tension, you may feel pain not only in your back but also in your neck, shoulders, arms, and legs. Tension-induced back pain is called *tension myositis syndrome*, or just simply TMS.

*Lower-Back Pain.* The primary causes of lower-back pain are many:

| | |
|---|---|
| Herniated disk | Lordosis |
| Poor posture | Kyphosis |
| Trauma resulting from injury (from sprains, strains, blows, or falls) | Spondylosis |
| | Foot problems (bunions, hammertoes, etc.) |
| Emotional stress | Arthritis (including osteoarthritis and ankylosing spondylitis) |
| Osteoporosis | |
| Fractures | Sports Injuries (multiple sprains, muscle pulls, shin splints, swelling, etc.) |
| Osteomalacia | |
| Scoliosis | |

*Muscle Cramps and Pain.* Certain nutritional deficiencies, postural problems, and dehydration can cause cramps and pains. If cramps and pains are diagnosed incorrectly—and they often *are*—the result can be persistent pain, poor healing, and sometimes unnecessary orthopedic surgery.

Two of the most prominent conditions associated with leg cramps are intermittent claudication and Buerger's disease.

*Intermittent Claudication* is generally associated with poor circulation, which may be caused by any number of disorders, such as: a blocked artery, blood vessel disease, diabetes, high blood cholesterol, or nutritional deficiencies.

*Buerger's Disease*, also known as "peripheral vascular disease," is a chronic inflammation of the blood vessels in a limb, usually a leg. The inflammation is caused by a clot formation, which prevents adequate circulation to the limb and, consequently, proper nourishment. As a result, the patient feels fatigued and has cold, painful limbs.

If an injury is involved, healing will be very slow because circulation is impaired. In advanced cases, ulceration and gangrene may set in. Buerger's disease is most common among young Jewish males.

*Bursitis.* Bursitis is an inflammation of the fluid filled sacs (bursa) found within joints, muscles, tendons and bones. The bursa reduce friction thus increasing muscular movement. X rays generally do not detect bursitis until the affected area is calcified.

*Carpal Tunnel Syndrome.* This is an arthritic condition that results when the median nerve in the wrist is compressed. Generally, the cause is the thickening of a ligament near the palm of the hand.

The symptoms of carpal tunnel syndrome may include:

• Impaired feeling and numbness in the hands.

• A tingling sensation radiating into the hands.

• Increased tingling and numbness when the wrist is flexed hard for 30 to 60 seconds.

• Shooting pains.

*Osteoporosis.* Osteoporosis, a weakening of the bones, is discussed in detail beginning on page 152.

*Sciatica.* Sciatica is a very painful condition that may possibly be caused by an inflammation of the sciatic nerve in the leg, or it may be a structural compensation for poor bone alignment. Although the precise cause is not known, sciatica seems to arise after an injury to this area of the leg.

*Thoracic Spine Disorders.* Most thoracic spine disorders involve vertebral disks T4-5, T5-6, and T6-7. When these vertebrae change positions, you may feel angina-like pain.

*Scoliosis.* Scoliosis, an abnormal curvature of the spine, can get progressively worse with age. Contrary to popular belief, this conditions does not necessarily stop with skeletal maturity. If left untreated, scoliosis can be very painful and can lead to complications such as heart and lung problems.

*Sprains.* Sprains and characterized by immediate swelling, pain, and in complicated sprains, possible discoloration.

*Shin Splints.* This term describes not a disease but any muscle pain in the shin bone (the tibia) between the knee and the ankle. Shin splints can result from improperly warming up before exercising, overusing lower-leg muscles, or wearing ill-fitting running shoes.

*Tennis Elbow.* Tennis elbow is a nonspecific, obscure pain that generally radiates to the outer side of the arm and forearm. When you consider that a tennis racquet travels about 300 miles an hour and then *slows down to 150 miles an hour* when it makes contact, you can see why this jolt to the elbow causes problems.

*Temporomandibular Joint Syndrome (TMJ).* Also known as "myofacial pain dysfunction," TMJ is a condition in which the upper and lower teeth do not meet properly. As a result of TMJ, you may feel any of the following symptoms: headaches, backaches, or bruxism (a clicking sound when you open and close your jaw).

See section on Dental and Oral Problems.

*Torticollis.* Torticollis, a contraction of the cervical muscles, is commonly called "wryneck."

## How Proper Nutrition Can Help

A good general suggestion for preventing musculoskeletal problems is to increase your use of green leafy vegetables. In addition, here are some other helpful suggestions for avoiding common disorders:

*For Athletes:* If you are athletic, follow a lactovegetarian diet with adequate protein and complex carbohydrates. Also, *Whole Foods Magazine* recommends supplementing your diet with avocados and unhydrogenated vegetable oils because they contain beta-sitosterol, which "can be converted to steroid hormones by the adrenal glands" ["Sports Nutrition," *Whole Foods Magazine*, July 1986, p. 18.] These steroid hormones can help reduce inflammation and increase healing from injuries.

*For TMJ Sufferers:* Eliminate foods that you find painful or difficult to chew—for example, apples, carrots, nuts, and bread. Instead, you will find the following foods more comfortable because they require less work on the part of your jaw muscles: nut butters (almond, cashew, peanut, etc.), apple sauce, soups, shredded carrots, or a blended salad (place fresh vegetables into a base of carrot and tomato juice and blend the mixture until it is completely liquefied). A diet of such foods will give your jaw muscles time to rest and recuperate!

*Osteoporosis.* A vegetarian diet tends to be lower in protein and phosphorus and requires less calcium. Therefore, there is a strong possibility that a vegetarian diet may lower the risk of osteoporosis.

## Supplements for Specific Conditions

If you suffer from any of the following musculoskeletal disorders, try these recommendations:

*For Backaches:* Take vitamins D and E in combination with calcium. These nutrients are important for proper formation and maintenance of your bones and as well as for nerve function.

*For Buerger's Disease:* Try high doses of vitamin E, 800–1200 iu.

*For Bursitis:* Take vitamin C, which has an anti-inflammatory effect. In the acute stages of bursitis, take vitamin E—as much as 1,200 iu a day. Also, vitamin $B_{12}$ injections help relieve bursitis.

*For Carpal Tunnel Syndrome:* Take 200 mg of vitamin $B_6$ three times a day. Also, whenever you take vitamin $B_6$ be sure to include EFAs and magnesium oxide.

*For Fractures:* For broken bones, take vitamins A, C, and D and pantothenic acid, calcium, phosporus, and potassium, all of which are required for forming new bone cells and the tissue fibers needed to bridge the two ends of a broken bone.

*For Lower-Back Pain:* Take 2,000 to 3,000 mg of vitamin C daily, particularly if you suffer pain from a slight disk deterioration. In addition, DL-Phenylalanine helps reduce lower-back pain, but it will take four to six weeks before you begin seeing results.

*For Leg Cramps:* A number of supplements are helpful in treating and preventing leg cramps:

1. *Vitamin E* (in doses of 2,000 iu a day) has been effective in providing relief from leg cramps, especially relief from nocturnal leg pain.

2. *Zinc* is beneficial in cases of severe vascular disease.

3. Calcium pangamate may help oxygen metabolism, according to studies conducted in the Soviet Union.

4. Other supplements that may help reduce and prevent cramping include:

| | |
|---|---|
| Vitamin B complex | Biotin |
| Vitamin C | Pantothenic acid |
| Vitamin D | Magnesium |
| EFAs | Phosphorus |

In addition, here are two recommendations that you may find very helpful:

*To Increase Strength and Endurance:* DMG, dimethylglycine, increases endurance, strength, and power, and it reduces lactic acid in muscle tissue. Octacosanol not only increases muscular strength and endurance, it increases reaction times and recovery time too, and it enhances performance of the neuromuscular system.

*To Reduce Injuries From Running:* Each day, take 1,000 mg of vitamin C for every 6 miles you run. The vitamin C will help protect you from collagen injuries in the joints and ligaments.

## Amino Acid Therapy

Take proline, an amino acid found in collagen (connective tissue) in conjunction with vitamin C. Proline may help repair muscle and tendon damage.

## Juice Therapy

Take Juice Therapy Formula #16 to strengthen your bone structure. (See the Appendix.)

## Aroma Therapy

Follow whichever of these suggestions applies to your condition:

*For Lower-Back Pain:* Essence of geranium.

*For Sciatica:* Essence of terebinth.

*For Spasms:* Essences of coriander, cypress, lavender, marjoram, and terebinth.

## Tissue Salts

Here are a number of tissue salt remedies that are effective in treating musculoskeletal disorders:

*For Sciatica:* Phosphate of iron, potassium phosphate, and magnesium phosphate.

*For Lower-Back Pain:* A combination of calcium flouride, calcium phosphate, potassium phosphate, and sodium chloride.

*For Inelasticity and Muscle Weakness:* Calcium flouride 6X.

*For Bone Disorders:* Calcium phosphate 6X.

*For Spasms, Neuralgia, and Sciatica:* Magnesium phosphate 6X.

*For Fibrositis and Muscular Pain:* A combination of phosphate or iron, potassium sulfate, and magnesium phosphate.

*For Cramping of the Legs and Feet:* A combination of calcium flouride, calcium phosphate, and magnesium phosphate.

*For Numbness and a "Sleeping Sensation" of the Legs:* Calcium phosphate.

## Acupuncture and Massage

Acupuncture has been found useful in treating TMJ.

Obviously, massage can be especially effective in dealing with musculoskeletal disorders. Here are some specific techniques that you may find helpful:

*For Lower-Back Pain:* Try deep pressure along zone #1 on your feet.

*For Muscle Trauma:* To avoid muscle atrophy and weakness, massage as soon as the swelling stops (generally about 48 hours after the injury). If massaging is delayed, scar tissue may form, and scar tissue may lead to further complications.

*For Thoracic Spine Disorders:* Manipulation of the spine is very helpful in cases of thoracic spine disorders.

*For Shin Splints:* Both before and after you exercise, try deep rhythmic pressure of the muscles of the lower leg.

*For Sprains:* Immediately after the sprain, try hydrotherapy. About 24 hours later, try range-of-motion exercises and gentle kneading. Use a counterirritant oil such as Olbas or Tiger Balm.

*For Sore Muscles:* Prepare a liniment by mixing: 1 tablespoon cayenne pepper, 1 tablespoon grated ginger and 1/2 cup Olive oil. Store this liniment in a warm place for one week, then rub the liniment into sore or aching muscles whenever necessary.

## The Edgar Cayce Muscle Treat Formula

Try this formula, which is specifically designed for backaches, bruises, strains, sprains, varicose veins, and sore muscles:

| | |
|---|---|
| Cola oil | Witch hazel |
| Mineral oil | Tincture benzoin |
| Olive oil | Sassafras oil |

## Exercise for Musculoskeletal Health

You can exercise away back pain and other disorders by following these recommendations:

*For Back Pain:* The best general exercises for preventing back pain include swimming, walking, and yoga. In addition, here are two other exercises you might try:

1. The Behind-the-Back Clasp. While sitting or standing, clasp your hands behind your neck. Now, without pulling or jerking, try to touch your elbows together. Hold this position for about 4 seconds, and repeat the exercise 10 times.

Although you will not be able to make your elbows touch, the exercise will be very helpful for your back.

2. Abdominal Exercises. Lie on your back in a fetal position with your hip and kneeds flexed. This strengthens your stomach muscles, thus helping to reduce back pain.

*For Buerger's Disease:* Do this exercise:

Lie on your back and elevate your legs to a 45-degree angle. Hold your legs in this position for 2 to 3 minutes. Your feet may turn white as blood flows away from them. Now sit on a bed and hang your feet off the edge for 5 to 10 minutes. Your feet will become red and flushed with blood. Next, lie flat on a soft surface and wrap your legs and feet to keep them warm.

Repeat these steps three or four times each session, and repeat the entire session three or four times each day.

*For Muscle Trauma:* As you saw earlier, it is important to *massage* as soon as possible after muscle trauma. Likewise, it is equally important to *exercise* as soon as possible after muscle trauma.

To increase your range of motion and reduce the potential for scar tissue to form, work out with swimming, very light weight-training exercises, yoga, and stretching exercises as soon as possible after a muscle injury.

*For Shin Splints:* Pay special attention to yoga and other stretching exercises. Also, be sure to warm up and cool down properly.

*For TMJ:* Do exercises that increase relaxation and improve posture, including hatha-yoga. In addition, do mouth exercises.

## Hydrotherapy

*For Back Pain:* Sponge with warm vinegar and water. Also, try taking a hot Epsom salt bath followed by very cold compresses or ice packs.

*For Muscle Spasms and Pain:* Alternate taking hot and cold showers.

*For a Sprained Ankle:* Try ice massages. Also, try cold compresses. Be sure to wrap the ankle afterward.

*For Sprains:* Apply locally either (1) ice or (2) sponges soaked with very cold water.

*For TMJ:* Use moist heat packs or ice massages around the jaw.

## Visualization Techniques for TMJ

To avoid the symptoms associated with TMJ, try this visualization technique:

Step 1: Find a quiet place where you will not be disturbed.

Step 2: Sit in a straight-back chair with your feet flat on the floor and hold your hands palms up on your knees.

Step 3: Close your eyes. Inhale and exhale long and slowly.

Step 4: As you exhale, visualize that you are actually exhaling out the stress and the tension from your body.

Step 5: Complete your visualization by (a) taking a long, deep breath, (b) slowly exhaling, and (c) gradually opening your eyes. Sit quietly for a few minutes as you become aware once again of your surroundings.

Step 6: Slowly begin to wiggle your fingers and toes.

Step 7: Rise only after you feel acclimated to your surroundings.

## How to Get Relief from Back Pain

Here are a number of items of interest concerning back pain:

*TNS Therapy.* TNS therapy has proved *very* helpful in relieving back pain, even in cases when all else has failed.

*Using X Rays to Diagnose Back Pain.* With few exceptions, X rays are *not* helpful in diagnosing back pain, unless the pain has lasted three months or more.

*Bed Rest for Back Pain.* Bed rest can shorten the duration of nonspecific back
pain. But the value of bed rest is limited. In comparison studies of people with
uncomplicated lower-back pain, *seven* days of rest proved no more helpful than *two*
days of rest. [*The New England Journal of Medicine*, Vol. 315, No. 17.]

*A Simple Remedy for a Compressed Disk.* When a compressed disk causes pain
and makes resting difficult, try this:

Lie on the floor with something padded beneath you. Rest your calves on a bed,
chair, or other support. Place a rolled towel under your neck during entire resting period.

*Sleeping Without Back Pain.* If you have back problems, your mattress must
provide stability. A water bed, therefore, is not a good choice for you. Instead, consider placing a plywood board between your mattress and box springs to provide extra
support and stability.

Futons, a Japanese mattress made of compressed cotton, are also highly recommended, because they can be as comfortable as a water bed and yet provide as much
stability as a very firm innerspring mattress.

Back sufferers often find it best to sleep on their sides with their knees bent.

*Sitting and Standing Without Back Pain.* Avoid soft, overstuffed chairs. Instead, sit on a hard chair, and make sure that your spine is pressed against the back of
the chair! Position a small stool in front of the chair and place one or both feet on this
stool. Reason: You will get relief if you keep one or both knees higher than your hips.

For driving, get a hard seat. Sit close enough to the wheel so that you do not need
to extend your legs to reach the pedals.

When you stand, make sure that your lower back is flat. When you work in a
standing position, use a footrest to help keep your back flat.

Women should avoid wearing high heels. Shoes with moderate heels cause less
back strain.

In addition, here are some items of interest concerning other musculoskeletal conditions:

*How to Get Relief From Leg Cramps.* Avoid wearing high-heel shoes, which
can cause leg cramps. Chelation therapy may be beneficial if other natural therapies
have not been effective. This technique involves intravenously feeding a specialized
chemical into the circulatory system to draw out heavy metals that cause hardening of
the arteries.

*How to Get Relief From Sciatica.* According to reports, daily injections of vitamin $B_{12}$ (1,000 mcg.) and vitamin $B_1$ (50 mg.) were instrumental in providing relief
from sciatica, although the reason why is unknown. Perhaps these nutrients reduce
nerve inflammation.

*How to Get Relief From TMJ.* If you suffer from TMJ, sleep lying on your back
rather than on your sides to prevent your jaw from being pushed to one side and thereby
adding stress to your jaw joints. Sleep on one flat pillow—not on several pillows and
not on thick pillows. A flat pillow will help your neck to curve less and relieve the
stress on the muscles of your jaw, neck, and upper back.

Also, be sure to avoid any habits or practices that may induce TMJ symptoms, for
example:

- Chewing gum.
- Biting your fingernails, lips, tongue, and cheeks.
- Clenching a pencil, pen, pipe, musical instrument, or any other object tightly between your teeth.
- Cradling a telephone, a violin, or any other object against your shoulder.

# 32

# Obesity

Did you know that . . .

- There are *over 28,000 diets* on public record?
- *65 percent* of Americans start new diets at least once a year?

Despite our apparent *mental* obsession with dieting, however, we Americans have no *physical* obsession with exercise and proper dietary habits. As a result, *obesity may be the greatest single health risk we face today.*

## The Dangers of Obesity

The bald fact is that obesity paves the way for other health problems. For example, obesity can create back problems. By weakening the *abdominal muscles*, obesity places greater stress on the *back muscles* to maintain an upright position. But this is not only health hazard created by obesity. Other potential problems include:

| | |
|---|---|
| Gallbladder disease | Hypertension |
| Arthritis | Reduced immune-system response |
| Diabetes | causing a greater risk of infection |
| Heart disease | |

## Some Basic Facts About Being Overweight

Learning some basic facts about obesity, nutrition, and dieting will provide you with the necessary background information you will need to begin a successful diet and to maintain a healthy weight.

- Poor nutrition is certainly the culprit in a majority of weight problems. True, big bones can account for obesity, and a thyroid condition (and other metabolic difficulties) can also account for obesity. Likewise, psychological factors and genetic factors, too, can account for obesity; but these are exceptions, they are not the rule!

• You may be overweight even though standard height-weight charts tell you that you are within the "normal range."

• As you age, the way your body holds fat will change, sometimes with dramatic results. For example, assume that a man has weighed 150 pounds for 20 years. Although he was not overweight 20 years ago, he may nonetheless be overweight today if his weight has been redistributed to his midsection.

• Generally speaking, if you are carrying 25 percent or more of your body weight in fat, then you are obese.

• Here is a quick rule of thumb for determining whether you are in a "safe" weight range: If you an adult male, your chest should be at least 5 inches larger than your waist. If you are an adult female, your chest should be 10 inches larger than your waist.

• For some very obese people, simply going on a long-term low-calorie diet may result in only a limited weight loss. Reason: Their metabolic rate may drop to "protect" them from starvation.

• According to recent research studies, "for many obese people, relatively small weight losses—say, only 10 percent of body weight—can correct a tendency toward diabetes or high blood pressure." Thus losing only 10 to 25 pounds can help avert major health risks. ["Research Lifts Blame From Many of the Obese," *New York Times*, March 24, 1987, Section C, p. 1.]

• As you lose weight, your body requires fewer calories. To continue losing weight at the same pace, therefore, you must lower your caloric intake. "For example, a moderately active female weighing 135 pounds can lose about a pound a week on a 1500-calorie diet. Once down to 124 pounds, however, she must consume no more than 1200 calories a day to maintain this rate of loss." ["Sad News for Dieters," *Working Together Bulletin*, Dartnell Corporation, 1986.]

## Dieting Traps

Just about any diet has the potential to help you lose weight, but your goal should always be to lose weight in a healthy, well-balanced manner *and then keep it off*!

Beware, however, of diet traps—diets that promote "unbalanced" weight-loss practices:

*Rigid Menus.* Few people follow diets that require strict adherence to rigid menus—at least, not for any reasonable length of time!

*Magic Formulas.* Diets that claim that certain foods will magically make fat disappear without any special calorie-control program are not worth following.

*"Promise You Everything" Diets.* Diets that "promise you everything"—losing large amounts *and* overnight at that—should arouse your natural suspicion. Remember: at the beginning of virtually *any* diet that restricts calories, carbohydrates, and salt, the weight you lose is *water*. Besides, studies show that the faster you lose weight, the more likely you are to regain it.

*Extreme Protein Diets.* Beware, too, of those diets that use excessively high or excessively low amounts of protein. Ingesting overly high levels of protein will increase your risk of many serious illnesses, including cancer and heart disease. Liquid high-protein diets tend to be too high in protein and too low in calories and may have side effects such as constipation, cramps, bad breath, and hair loss.

When your diet is too low in protein, your body may utilize the protein from your own organs and muscles.

*Diets Under 1,000 Calories.* When you cut your caloric intake very suddenly, your body may reduce the number of calories it burns. Thus you may follow a low-calorie diet and still not lose weight. In general, the more extreme a diet appears, the less likely it is to help you lose weight and then keep weight off.

*Fasting.* Fasting can be a very powerful healing tool, but it is not effective as part of a weight-control program. The two most important dietary factors in an effective weight-loss program are (1) choosing foods properly and (2) eating moderately. Fasting does not help you practice either one!

There are other reasons why fasting is not a good dieting tool. Unsupervised long fasts can cause kidney failure, blood-pH problems, liver malfunction, electrolyte depletion, a drop in intestinal absorption of nutrients, and a reduction in the digestive enzyme level in the stomach and intestines.

## One Calorie Does Not Always Equal One Calorie

Are all calories equal? Does it matter whether you intake one calorie from a *fat* or one calorie from a *carbohydrate*?

For years, some experts argued that all calories *are* equal: x calories from one food must equal x calories from any other food. But recent research shows otherwise.

According to Dr. Elliott Danforth of the University of Vermont, "only about one percent of ingested carbohydrates end up as body fat," as opposed to 2.5 percent for ingested fats. Therefore, one calorie from a fat is *less efficient* for weight loss than one calorie from a starch. As a result, "simply switching from a high-fat diet to one high in carbohydrates, without actually lowering total caloric intake, can result in a net caloric loss to the body," ["Research Lifts Blame From Many of the Obese," *The New York Times*, March 24, 1987, Section C, p. 6.]

## General Dieting Tips to Lose Weight Efficiently

To lose weight in the most efficient, healthy way, follow these dieting tips:

• Adopt a vegetarian diet, which has a lower intake of fat. Also, because a vegetarian diet is high in fiber and uses lots of low-calorie vegetables, you will generally satisfy your feelings of hunger more fully on a vegetarian diet.

• Every morning, establish a meal plan for the day to help you avoid "spontaneous eating." For example, if you schedule lunch for 1:00 p.m., then stick to your plan!

• Keep a diary of what you eat. Despite the fact that you are dieting, you will be eating large amounts of food. However, it will probably *seem* as if you are eating very small amounts. Your diary will encourage you by providing otherwise!

• Each day, drink as much as 8 glasses of fluids—water, broth, or cleansing herbal teas. You will reduce your hunger pangs and at the same time cleanse your body of toxic substances that gather as you burn body fat.

• Divide your total caloric intake among six very small meals a day. Spreading meals will help you avoid sweets and sugary snacks between meals. It will also reduce the outpouring of insulin that accompanies large meals and that may increase body fat.

• Eat slowly. Avoid reading or watching TV while you eat. Sit down comfortably and concentrate on what you are doing.

• Do not keep snacks in your house, even if you keep them "for friends who drop by."

• To lose more weight, eat your largest meals earlier in the day. People lose less weight and at a slower pace when they ₋at large evening meals.

• Do not use food as a reward.

• Exercise regularly!

• Use anything you can to help motivate yourself to stick to your diet—for example, pictures of yourself when you were thinner, smaller-size clothing, or anything else that get results.

• If you have a small frame and your ideal weight is between 100 and 130 pounds, do not lose more than 2 pounds a week. If you have a larger frame and your ideal weight is over 130 pounds, do not lose more than 3 pounds a week.

## Food Tips to Help You Lose Weight Efficiently

To lose weight in the most efficient way, follow these specific food recommendations:

• Eat a variety of fresh, unrefined, unprocessed foods.

• Include lots of high-fiber foods and complex carbohydrates, such as fresh fruits, vegetables, whole grains, and beans. As much as 30 percent of the calories found in complex carbohydrates are not absorbed and will pass through your body without adding to your caloric intake! Because you tend to feel more satisfied after meals with a smaller caloric intake, you will lose weight slowly and steadily.

• Be sure to avoid:

| | |
|---|---|
| High-calorie foods | Alcohol |
| Foods with too much saturated fat | Too much sodium |
| Refined white sugar and brown sugar (and all foods that contain them) | Gravies and heavy sauces |
| | Foods that are too hot or too cold |

• Also avoid drinking fluids excessively with your meals and eating when you are under great stress.

• Broil, steam, or bake all foods that you do not eat raw. Do not add oil or butter.

• Use moderate amounts of protein and little or no saturated fats.

• Prepare small portions.

• Bake several potatoes and keep them in the refrigerator for snacks. Then, when you are hungry, cut a potato in half and eat it with a tablespoon of yogurt.

• If you use sweeteners such as honey and maple syrup, use them in moderation.

• If you use butter, dilute it half-and-half with sunflower oil.

• If you use dairy products, goat's milk is better than cow's milk.

## A Word About Sweeteners

Artificial sweeteners help you to lose weight—right? Wrong!

As a result of many research studies, there is conclusive evidence to show that artificial sweeteners are ineffective for weight control or weight loss. For example, in one survey of more than 78,000 women, those "who used artificial sweeteners were more likely to gain weight than women who didn't. They also gained weight faster, regardless of the weight they were to begin with." [Karen MacNeil, "Diet Soft Drinks: Too Good to Be True?" *The New York Times*, February 4, 1987, Section C, p. 3.]

And Aspartame, a brand name for one sweetener, "may produce a 'residual hunger' that leads to increased food consumption" and "may send ambiguous signals to the brain, resulting in a loss of control over appetite"! [Karen MacNeil, "Diet Soft Drinks: Too Good to Be True?" *The New York Times*, February 4, 1987, Section C, p. 3.]

## Some Helpful Supplements for Weight Loss

Here are three supplements that are especially helpful in a weight-control program:

*Bioflavonoids.* When you lose a lot of weight, you also lose a layer of padding, namely, *fat*. Without this layer of fat, which once protected the capillaries, you may experience skin bruising. Bioflavonoid supplementation will help to strengthen your capillaries and prevent skin bruising, but it may take as long as three months to see results.

*Choline and Methionine.* Choline transports fat for use as a body fuel. To reduce your body fat while increasing your energy reserves, take choline together with methionine.

*Inositol.* To control your appetite and maintain your glucose levels, supplement with inositol.

## Amino Acid Therapy

Amino acid supplementation can be very helpful in weight loss and weight control. At the same time, however, amino acid supplementation can be easily abused by someone with a compulsive eating pattern.

Use the following amino acids only as part of a well-balanced, nutritionally sound weight-loss program:

*Arginine and Ornithine.* These nonessential amino acids increase the secretion of human growth hormone (HGH), which may cause the body to burn up fat reserves. They also promote muscle tone.

*Leucine, Isoleucine, and Baline.* These three amino acids are used directly by muscle tissue as a source of energy. For best results, take all three together.

*Carnitine.* Carnitine helps the body use its fat reserves for fuel. It also stimulates and maintains the adrenal gland.

*D,L-Phenylalanine and L-Tyrosine.* These two amino acids are appetite suppressants and antidepressants. They release chemicals that tell your brain that your stomach is full, even if you haven't eaten. You should take vitamin $B_6$, a natural diuretic, whenever you take L-Tyrosine because Vitamin $B_6$ is essential to the proper functioning of this amino acid.

CAUTION: Methionine must be taken along with vitamin $B_6$ to inhibit the synthesis of homocysteine, which promotes plaque deposits in the arteries.

## Juice Therapy

Unless you are on a supervised juice therapy program, you should avoid most fruit and vegetables juices while you are following a weight-loss program. Many dieters drink large quantities of juices because they consider juices lower in calories. However, many juices may actually be *higher* in calories; at the same time, juices do not have the benefit of fiber.

Here is one juice formula that you *will* find helpful: Add to a 16-ounce glass of combined carrot, beet, and apple juices one teaspoon of bee pollen. This formula will help support your glandular function.

## Herbs That Contribute to Your Weight Loss

Here are some herbs that can help you lose weight:

• To reduce your appetite and lower the fat levels stored in your body, before each meal drink a tea made from *chickweed, burdock root, and nettle.*

• Place a teaspoon of powdered *flaxseed or psyllium seed husks* in a cup of warm water and drink this mixture to reduce your craving for food.

• In modern China, herbalists still use these old remedies to help suppress the appetite: *Chinese apricots, Chinese quince, and dried peony root.*

## Massage

Use circular and deep rhythmic pressure on both earlobes. See the Appendix.

## Exercise to Lose Weight

Exercise burns up calories while you exercise *and* for several hours afterward; and exercise replaces fat with lean muscle tissue. An added benefit is that lean muscle tissue, in turn, allows you to increase your calories without gaining weight. As a result, exercise—especially aerobic exercise—is especially valuable in any weight-loss program.

## Hydrotherapy

To increase your glandular function, try cool full-body baths or sitz baths.

## Emotional Factors

Radical changes in eating and exercise patterns are very difficult—nearly impossible—to achieve in less than five or six months. The reason is simple: Old habits and long-established patterns are hard to break even over a period of time.

Many people react to tension by overeating. If you are to be successful in losing weight and maintaining a normal, healthy weight, you must address the cause of your tension. You must learn to control your responses to tension, rather than be a victim of stressful, tense situations.

## Motivate Yourself!

Let's face it, if you are *not* sufficiently motivated, you will not lose weight. You must motivate yourself to a great degree, but you can also rely on others for added support, of course. Learn to rely on your family, friends and co-workers for help in keeping to your weight-loss program. Better yet, consider joining a weight-loss support group.

You must *actively* work to keep your motivation high. Here are a number of *do*s and *don't*s to keep your motivation level at its peak:

1. *Do* ask your family and friends not to bring you food, snacks, treats, or anything else that can undermine your program. Control your home environment so that you will be able to avoid factors that foster overeating, such as easy access to food, food in full view, and vulnerability to food cues.

2. *Do* learn to choose the proper foods in restaurants, even though friends and associates may be eating foods that are not on your diet.

3. In restaurants, *don't* accept food that has not been prepared as you requested. Don't be shy; talk to the waiter or waitress or, if necessary, the maitre d'.

4. *Don't* allow friends or acquaintances to sabotage your efforts (innocently or otherwise) by saying, for example, "You look fine—you don't really need to lose weight." You will *want* to agree, of course, but you must stand firm. Do not give in to such temptation.

5. *Don't* be embarrassed at parties or other social functions when you are asked why you are not eating certain foods. Answer truthfully. There is no shame in dieting!

6. *Don't* be "forced" into eating something by comments such as "Try this—I just cooked it." Or "It's only a little piece—it won't hurt you." Politely decline.

7. *Do* avoid watching tempting food commercials. Change the channel!

8. *Do* learn to make eating a wonderful experience. After all, it *is*.

## Visualization Techniques

Your self-image plays an important role in weight loss. Try to visualize yourself in two distinct pictures: one is the "before" picture, the how-overweight you; the other is the "after" picture, the new, slimmer, thinner you. Use the "before" picture to convince yourself of the need to lose weight. Use the "after" picture to keep your goal in mind and for continued encouragement and motivation.

Try this visualization technique: Find a quiet place where you will not be disturbed. Sit in a straight-back chair with both feet flat on the floor and hold your hands, palms up, on your knees. Close your eyes. Inhale and exhale long and slowly. As you exhale, visualize your "after" picture, what you will look like after you have reached your weight-loss goals.

Complete your visualization by (a) taking a long, deep breath, (b) slowly exhaling, and (c) gradually opening your eyes. Sit quietly for a few minutes as you become aware once again of your surroundings. Slowly begin to wiggle your fingers and toes. Rise only after you feel acclimated to your surroundings.

# 33

# Osteoporosis

As its name implies, *osteoporosis* describes a thinning and porosity of the bones. It is a particularly disabling disease because thin, porous bones are weak and, are more likely to break—even as a result of normal, everyday activities.

## Women Are Especially Susceptible

Osteoporosis affects women more often than men, although the reasons why are not clear. In fact, the two conditions that plague menopausal women most are heart disease and osteoporosis.

Perhaps women are more susceptible to osteoporosis because:

- They have less bone mass than men have.
- They have smaller bones and thus have less calcium.
- Women live longer than men and therefore have more time to lose the calcium in their bones.
- Women engage in weight-bearing exercises less often than men do (weight-bearing exercises promote calcium retention and increase bone mass).

## Common Causes

Osteoporosis can result from a number of causes, including:

- A postmenopausal deficiency of the hormone estrogen.
- A calcium deficiency, which might simply be the result of not eating enough high-calcium foods.
- A deficiency in the enzyme lactase, which is needed to digest milk sugar. This deficiency is known to be more common among people suffering from osteoporosis.

• Caffeine use. Studies show that drinking coffe increases calcium loss. To aggravate this condition further, people who ingest large amounts of caffeine each day also generally eat fewer high-calcium foods. [*Journal of Laboratory and Clinical Medicine*, January 1982.]

• Smoking cigarettes. Smoking may cause a chain reaction in women. Women who smoke may have less estrogen in their bodies. Reason: They have about 50 percent more of an enzyme that reduces the amount of estrogen. The reduced amount of estrogen brings on menopause earlier, and menopause, in turn, radically speeds up bone loss.

The net result of this chain reaction is that smoking can contribute to osteoporisis in women.

• Consuming alcoholic beverages.

• Physical inactivity. Lack of exercise can cause a loss in bone calcium and a decreased ability to replace the lost calcium.

• A vitamin C deficiency. The body's bone-forming cells, called "osteoblasts," use vitamin C to make the structural support for bone minerals.

• Abnormal parathyroid activity. When your dietary intake of phosphorus is too high, the parathyroid may be stimulated, causing the removal of calcium from the bones. Thus some nutritionists suspect that meat (which is high in phosphorus and low in calcium) and highly refined sugar products contribute to osteoporosis.

## Good Nutrition Thwarts Osteoporosis

Following a sound nutrition program can help you build strong bones and fight off the possibility of osteoporosis.

Avoid eating excessive amounts of protein, especially beef and other meats. Excessive protein results in a loss of calcium. Calcium may be lost when sulfur-containing amino acids are metabolized. Meat is high in sulfur-containing amino acids and would contribute to this loss of calcium.

Not surprisingly, vegetarians in their 70s and 80s generally have a greater bone mass and a lower incidence of osteoporosis than meat-eaters in their 60s. [*American Journal of Clinical Nutrition*, June 1972. *Journal of the American Dietetic Association*, February 1980.]

Increase your intake of diary products. Yogurt, kefir, buttermilk, and other cultured dairy products are best. Also, use high-mineral foods, which include:

| | |
|---|---|
| Sea vegetables | Green vegetables |
| Raw, unsalted nuts and seeds | Cabbage |
| Whole grains | Strawberries, blueberries, and raspberries |

## Your Supplementation Program

Because calcium increases bone density, be sure to include calcium lactate or calcium carbonate in your daily diet. [*New England Journal of Medicine*, August 13, 1981.] Studies show that calcium can even increase bone density in the elderly. [*American Journal of Clinical Nutrition.*]

Here is an excellent daily supplementation for you:

Vitamin $B_{12}$

Vitamin C (1,000 mg.)

Vitamin D (400 iu)

Vitamin E (600 iu)

Copper

Fluoride

Magnesium chloride (400 mg.)

Phosphorus

Calcium lactate or calcium carbonate
(for premenopausal women, 1,000 mg.;
for postmenopausal women, 1,500 mg.)

A multiple trace-mineral supplement

Silica tablets

Alfalfa tablets

Betain HCL (take 1-2 tablets
with water after each meal)

## Herbs, Too, Can Help

Use the following herbs as part of your prevention program:

Horsetail       Parsley

Nettle          Alfalfa

Comfrey         Mullein

## Exercise

Studies offer conclusive evidence that regular exercise increases mineral bone mass. [*Physician and Sports Medicine*, March 1982.] Not exercising certainly accelerates the thinning of bones. Therefore, a regular exercise program is extremely valuable in preventing osteoporosis.

The most appropriate exercises include walking, running, tennis, calisthenics, and all weight-bearing exercises.

## Tissue Salts

Try calcium fluoride 6X as an additional source of calcium.

# 34

# Pain

Consider pain as nature's signal that something is wrong. Because pain has a specific purpose, *to warn you*, you should never ignore pain. Perhaps even worse, if you attempt to deaden the pain or eliminate it in an effort to avoid discomfort, you may aggravate the cause of the pain and allow the pain to spread. Instead, you must discover the underlying cause of the pain and treat the cause, not simply the symptoms.

## The Role of Good Nutrition

Research studies show that nutrition can directly affect how you perceive pain. Specifically, chronic pain can be relieved by these essential amino acids: leucine, phenylalanine and tryptophan.

These amino acids function as messengers, relaxing nerve cells in the brain that send pain information. As the level of these amino acids increases, the body's level of serotonin also increases, and serotonin is the most important messenger for relieving pain.

As a result, you can benefit from these suggestions:

• To increase your threshold for pain, follow a diet high in carbohydrates, low in fats, and low in proteins.

• For an even greater increase in your pain threshold, add to the above diet 3 grams of L-Tryptophan.

• Reduce your corn intake. Studies show that people who followed corn-rich diets had a lower tolerance for pain, perhaps because corn is low in L-Tryptophan.

- Include these Tryptophan-rich foods in your diet:

| | |
|---|---|
| Soybeans and soy protein | Green leafy vegetables |
| Cottage cheese | Yogurt |
| Mixed nuts | Brown rice |
| Baked beans (sugar-free) | Raw, unsalted pumpkin and sesame seeds |
| Lentils | Avocados |
| Bananas | Pineapples |

- Include these Phenylalanine-rich foods in your diet: nuts, soybeans, and other beans.

- Except for the protein foods listed above, avoid concentrated proteins like meat, fish, eggs, or poultry in a pain-control program. These foods may reduce Tryptophan levels and serotonin levels. Instead, eat complex carbohydrates, which are highly recommended.

## Effective Supplements

Here are some supplements that are especially effective in a pain-control program:

*L-Tryptophan, Niacin, and Vitamin B_6.* The combination of these three supplements is very helpful for pain relief because together they increase the serotonin level in the body.

*D,L-Phenylalanine (DLPA).* Phenylalanine supplements are anti-inflammatory agents and are helpful in reducing *chronic* pain. They are, however, of limited value in reducing *acute* pain, that is, pain lasting just a few hours.

DLPA can successfully reduce pain associated with:

| | |
|---|---|
| Arthritis | Migraine headaches |
| Gout | Neuralgia resulting from shingles |
| Ankylosing spondylitis | Cervical spondylosis |
| Systemic lupus | Lumbar fusion |
| Erythematosis | Postlaminectomy |
| Bursitis | Menses |

To avoid competition with other amino acids, take DLPA 1½ to 2 hours before meals.

*CAUTIONS:* If you suffer from high blood pressure or use antidepressants that inhibit monoamine oxidase (MAO), be extremely careful when taking DLPA. If you do take DLPA, take it within 5 or 10 minutes after meals.

Under *no* circumstances should you take DLPA if you are pregnant, or if you suffer from phenylketonurics (PKU), a rare genetic disorder which makes it impossible for the body to process DLPA.

## Your Supplementation Program

Include the following in your daily supplementation program: Leucine, D,L-Phenylalanine (see previous CAUTIONS), L-Tryptophan, Niacin, Vitamin B_6.

## Hot Pepper for Pain Relief

For pain relief, use extract of hot pepper. For centuries, this remedy has been used effectively for pain relief, but the reason for its effectiveness was discovered only a few years ago:

> Recently scientists have found evidence that capsaicin, the pungent ingredient in hot peppers, acts against pain. . . . Capsaicin . . . selectively stimulates and then blocks some nerve fibers that end in the skin and mucous membranes. ["Science Watch," *The New York Times*, June 28, 1983, p. 00.]

## Aroma Therapy

Try essence of cloves for general pain relief. Also, to reduce the minor pains associated with sprains, strains, and arthritis, combine capsicum, camphor, turpentine, and pine oils and apply the mixture externally.

## Acupressure and Massage

For head and neck pain, use both thumbs to apply circular rhythmic pressure at the base of the skull. For jaw pain, see Chart #0 on page 00.

## Exercise

To soothe stiff joints and to help sprains and strains to heal, try range-of-motion exercises, *unless* swelling or inflammation is present.

## Also of Interest

*Biofeedback and Acupuncture.* These two techniques are effective in reducing pain. Moreover, biofeedback and acupuncture have been found effective in reducing the chronic pain associated with depression.

*Self-Hypnosis.* Dr. Candice Erickson of New York's Columbia Presbyterian Medical Center teaches children to use self-hypnosis to control pain in conditions ranging from sickle-cell anemia to leukemia. According to Dr. Erickson, hypnosis is "an altered state of consciousness in which a person is so focused, concentrated and relaxed that he excludes other stimuli." Because the *children* control the hypnosis, not a *hypnotherapist*, "Hypnosis gives children a sense of mastery over their own illness." [Carol Lawson, "Sick Children Learn Self-Hypnotism to Fight Pain, *The New York Times*, September 7, 1985, p. 00.]

*The Role of Endorphins.* Endorphins are natural opiate-like substances found in the brain. One of the functions of endorphins is to control pain. Interestingly, studies show that natural healing processes such as acupuncture and visualization can raise the body's level of endorphins. Even jogging and listening to music can effect endorphin levels.

# 35

# Pregnancy

During pregnancy, your body undergoes many natural changes. Although the changes *are* "natural," they may not feel natural to you. In fact, some may feel rather strange, especially if this is your first pregnancy.

As a result of the changes your body will undergo, you may experience a number of discomforts or physical difficulties. Even though they may be harmless, perfectly natural feelings, you should understand them nonetheless.

For example, you may feel fatigue during the first few months of pregnancy. Even though you may sleep a few hours more than is usual for you, you may still feel tired. By the fourth or fifth month, the feeling of fatigue may lessen or it may disappear. On the other hand, it may return later.

Remember, such feelings are perfectly natural!

## Some Common Discomforts

In addition to feeling fatigued, you may experience some of the following common physical difficulties and discomforts associated with pregnancy:

| | |
|---|---|
| Backaches | Pain in the round ligaments (the ligaments |
| Bleeding gums | that hold the uterus in place) |
| Constipation | Sciatic pain |
| Edema | Vaginal bleeding |
| Heartburn | Vaginal discharge |
| Hemmorhoids | Vaginal pressure and tingling |
| Leg cramps | Varicose veins |
| Morning sickness | |

Let's take a closer look at some of these discomforts.

*Backaches.* You are less likely to suffer from backaches if you practiced good posture and exercised regularly before pregnancy. If backaches do develop, you should consider:

- Take a class in postural alignment.
- Wear a good support bra.
- Use a firmer mattress or place a sheet of plywood under your present mattress for added back support.

*Bleeding Gums.* You are more likely to have bleeding gums during pregnancy. Hormone changes cause the mucous membranes to soften and at the same time increase the blood supply. Your gums are very sensitive to these changes and may react by bleeding.

*Constipation.* Constipation may result from natural hormonal changes and from the increased size of the uterus during pregnancy. To counteract constipation, exercise regularly. Also, eat high-fiber foods (fresh fruits and vegetables) and whole grains, and drink plenty of liquids.

*Edema.* *Edema* means "swelling." During pregnancy, body tissues may retain fluids, and these retained fluids cause swelling. Swelling is also caused by sluggish circulation, which results from the extra weight carried in the uterus. Standing or sitting in one place for too long a time will aggravate swelling.

To reduce the effects of edema, elevate your legs. Also, try lying on your left side to take the weight off your inferior vena cava, one of the major veins in the body.

Although edema is uncomfortable, it is not usually a health threat so long as your blood pressure is normal and you have no protein in your urine (your physician should check for protein in the urine).

*Heartburn.* Heartburn, which is especially common during the last few months of pregnancy, is the result of this brief chain reaction:

In the later months, the body level of the hormone progesterone increases. Increases in this hormone cause the esophagus muscles to relax. As the esophagus muscles relax, the contents of the stomach may back up, causing heartburn.

To relieve the feeling of heartburn, try these remedies:

- Take small sips of peppermint tea or ginger tea.
- Avoid foods that you find cause heartburn.
- At bedtime, place an extra pillow under your neck or your upper-back area, or elevate your bed.

*Hemorrhoids.* Common during pregnancy, hemorrhoids are usually aggravated by constipation and forced bowel movements. Remedy: Add lots of high-fiber foods to your diet.

*Leg Cramps.* In the later months, the expanded uterus places pressure on the nerves that run from the pelvis to the lower legs. Often, the result of this pressure is leg cramps.

To relieve leg cramps, increase your calcium supplementation and do exercises specifically intended to stretch out the muscles that cramp and to increase the general circulation to that area. See "Stretching Exercises That Relieve Cramps" beginning on page 164.

*Morning Sickness.* To avoid morning sickness, the feeling of nausea or vomiting common during the first three months of pregnancy, follow these tips:

1. Eat small amounts of food every 1 or 2 hours.

2. Avoid greasy foods, fatty foods, and foods with very strong tastes and odors.

3. Before bedtime, eat a high-protein snack such as yogurt or buttermilk for extra nourishment for the early-morning hours the next day.

A study presented at the Tenth World Congress on Gynecology in 1982 indicates "a possible relationship between nausea in pregnancy and impaired liver function." As a result, the therapies used to treat liver disease might be effective in treating morning sickness. Also, according to this study "women with allergies and gastritis and those who suffered side effects from oral contraceptives were much more likely to suffer from nausea when pregnant." [*New York Times*, October 24, 1982, p. 24.]

*Pain in the Round Ligaments.* As the uterus enlarges, the round ligaments stretch and often cramp, causing pain that you may feel either on one side or on both sides of the abdomen. To relieve this discomfort, try applying a heat message. Also, do the "knee-to-chest stretch" exercise described on page 164.

*Sciatic Pain.* When the fetus places pressure on the sciatic nerve, you will surely feel pain in the area. For relief from sciatic pain, apply a moist heating pad or a moist warm towel to the area. Also, see "Stretching Exercises That Relieve Cramps" on page 164.

*Vaginal Bleeding.* Vaginal bleeding during pregnancy is common and is usually no cause for concern. Called "spotting" or "staining," bleeding is especially common at the time of the first two missed menstrual periods. For some women, however, staining may take place throughout the pregnancy. Of course, you should report any abnormal bleeding to your physician.

*Vaginal Discharge.* During pregnancy, a pale, mucus-like discharge is normal—in fact, it is healthy, because it will help lubricate the vagina and ease delivery.

*Vaginal Pressure and Tingling.* As the fetus moves, you may feel the sensation of pressure of tingling, especially toward the end of pregnancy.

*Varicose Veins.* Varicose veins, which may appear in the legs and around the vulva, will become worse unless the condition is treated. To prevent varicose veins, or to treat them once they appear, wear good support stockings throughout your pregnancy.

## What About Breast-Feeding?

Breast-feeding protects infants from eczema, although the underlying reasons *why* it protects is not known. Also, studies show that breast-feeding protects infants from allergies.

A vegetarian diet is highly recommended for women who plan to breast-feed. Research studies show that vegetarian women have fewer pollutants, pesticide residues, and other chemicals that build up in animal fat—substances that may be passed on through breast-feeding.

## Nutrition During Pregnancy

Good nutrition plays an exceptionally important role during pregnancy and affects the health of both mother and child. Research studies offer conclusive evidence that pregnant women who have poor nutritional habits are more likely to undergo premature labor than women who followed healthy diets throughout pregnancy. Specific topics concerning nutrition for pregnant women are discussed next.

## Increased Nutritional Requirements

Pregnant women have an increased requirement for certain nutrients:

*Calories.* A woman who does *not* change her level of activity during pregnancy will require an additional 300 to 500 calories a day. But most authorities agree that a pregnant woman should not need more than 2,200 calories a day.

According to Dr. Myron Winiol, Director of the Institute of Human Nutrition at Columbia University's College of Physicians and Surgeons, "A good rule of thumb is that a woman should reach about 120 percent of her ideal weight at the end of pregnancy." [*New York Sunday News*, September 28, 1986, p. 12.]

*Protein.* Protein is essential for building fetal tissue, especially the brain and the placenta. If you plan to breast-feed, add 20 grams of protein to your daily nutritional requirements.

*Iron.* During pregnancy, your blood will require more iron, and the fetus, too, will need more iron as a reserve for the first few months of life. Be sure to eat plenty of these iron-rich foods: green leafy vegetables, dried beans and blackstrap molasses.

Many nutritionists recommend that women in their second and third trimesters supplement their diets with 30 to 60 milligrams of iron daily.

*B Vitamins.* The B vitamins, especially folic acid and pyridoxine, are very important nutrients during pregnancy. Folic acid is essential for producing protein in the early months of pregnancy.

*Salt.* Although some physicians recommend lowering salt intake during pregnancy in an effort to reduce swelling and water retention, be sure *not* to lower your daily salt intake below 2,000 milligrams.

*Miscellaneous.* Other major nutrients needed during pregnancy are calcium, vitamin A, and vitamin C. Also, be sure to drink more fluids each day.

## What to Avoid

Certain substances are strictly taboo for pregnant women, including these:

*Alcohol.* Drinking even moderate amounts of alcohol can cut off oxygen to the fetus, and consistent drinking can permanently injure the child's brain and nervous system. In addition, consuming large quantities of alcohol immediately after fertilization may cause genetic abnormalities and result in miscarriage.

Among the birth defects caused by drinking alcohol during pregnancy are:

| | |
|---|---|
| Intellectual handicaps | Heart murmurs |
| Low birth weight | Ear disorders |
| Facial deformities | Skeletal problems |

*Coffee.* In one study of 16 pregnant women, all of whom drank 8 or more cups of coffee a day, the reported results were disastrous: Only *1* woman went through labor and childbirth without complications. The other 15 pregnancies ended in spontaneous abortion, stillbirth, or premature birth.

The message is clear. During pregnancy, be sure to avoid drinking coffee.

*Soft Cheeses.* Pregnant women are well advised to avoid soft cheeses such as Liederkranz, Brie, and Camembert. The reason is that pregnant women may be more susceptible to a certain widespread bacterium (*Listeria monocytogenes*) found more often in soft cheeses than in hard cheeses. Although this bacterium may cause no harm to others, pregnant women run a higher risk of susceptibility.

*Marijuana.* Studies show that pregnant women who smoked marijuana three or more times a week delivered babies at lower birth weights than mothers who did not use marijuana. In fact, the birth weights of babies of marijuana-smoking mothers were even lower than the weights of babies of cigarette-smoking mothers.

## Nutritional Remedies for Specific Ailments

Pregnant women can use sound nutritional therapies to treat some common ailments:

*Constipation.* To treat constipation, pregnant women should follow these recommendations:

- Avoid eating:

Hard-boiled eggs

Boiled milk

Processed foods

Products with refined flour (white bread, pizza dough, and so on)

Foods that contain tannin (such as red wine, tea, cocoa, peppermint tea, and cloves)

Foods that absorb moisture (celery, radishes, carrots, and lettuce, for example)

- Instead, use foods that have a slight laxative effect:

Strawberries

Protein-aide brand sesame seeds (recommended because they are hulled without any chemicals)

Raw spinach

Watermelon

[Betty Kamen, "Pregnancy Ailments," *Health & Diet Times*, April/May 1982, p. 12.]

*Morning Sickness.* To avoid morning sickness, follow these three suggestions:
1. Drink plenty of fluids.
2. Alternately eat low-protein meals and high-protein snacks.
3. Reduce your intake of animal protein and high-fat and spicy foods.

## Special Supplements for Pregnant Women

Supplementation is of great value during pregnancy, especially for women suffering from morning sickness. Here are the supplements that are most effective for pregnant women:

*Vitamin B₆ and Magnesium:* For morning sickness, especially to avoid the nausea associated with morning sickness, take 200 milligrams of vitamin $B_6$ daily. Also, take vitamins K and C to reduce the effects of morning sickness. [*American Journal of Obstetrics and Gynecology,* August 1952.]

In addition, when taken with magnesium, vitamin $B_6$ is helpful in treating preeclampsia.

*Octacosanol:* This supplement reduces the risk of spontaneous abortion.

*L-Tryptophan:* L-Tryptophan is helpful in relieving postpartum depression. Postpartum depression is discussed in greater detail on page 165.

*Vitamin C and Iron:* Pregnant women need both vitamin C and iron: For optimal formation of hemoglobin, 500 milligrams of vitamin C will "balance" 100 milligrams of iron. In any case, pregnant women need at least 300 milligrams of vitamin C daily to prevent scurvy. [W. H. Birkenhager, in a letter to *The Lancet,* October 13, 1973, p. 859.]

## Juice Therapy

According to N. W. Walker, drinking one pint of carrot juice a day may help reduce the possibility of puerperal sepsis at childbirth. [N. W. Walker, *Raw Vegetable Juices,* New York, Pyramid Books, 1976, p. 00.]

## Effective Herbs During Pregnancy

During pregnancy, try red raspberry leaf tea. Because red raspberry leaf is high in calcium and magnesium, this tea should help keep you strong and healthy.

Among the specific uses of herbs during pregnancy are the following:

*For Anemia:* Nettle, borage, clover, alfalfa, and red raspberry.

*For Increased Milk Flow in Breast-Feeding:* Marsh mallow root, fennel seed, borage, and anise.

*For Nausea:* According to *The Lancet,* powdered ginger root (in capsule form) can be very effective for nausea. [*The Lancet,* March 20, 1982.] In addition, raspberry leaves, apple peels, blackberries, mint, and peach leaves can also be useful in fighting off nausea.

*To Aid in Delivery:* Take squaw vine during the last two weeks of your pregnancy. Also, try these herbs: lavender, basil, nutmeg, and red raspberry leaves.

*To Expel the Placenta:* Use pennyroyal, chamomile, and basil.

*To Stop Excess Bleeding:* Take capsicum, shepherd's purse, yarrow, and nettle.

*For Jaundice:* Take alfalfa and red raspberry leaves.

NOTE: Avoid using pennyroyal and rue during pregnancy.

## Aroma Therapy

Certain essences are very effective natural health aids for pregnant women and breast-feeding mothers. Note the following:

*To Help Induce Labor:* To stimulate uterine contractions and therefore help produce quick, less-painful births, try: oil of jasmine, juniper, and pennyroyal. Apply these essences as compresses to the lower abdomen, or if you wish, simply massage them into the lower-back area.

*To Increase Milk Flow:* Use estrogen-like substances, such as fennel oil.
*To Prepare for Childbirth:* Try oil of clove and oil of sage.

## Acupressure and Massage

Try kneading and gentle circular rhythmic pressure. When you are pregnant, never lie facedown for a massage.

## Exercise Moderately

As long as your pregnancy is normal and free of complications, you can certainly benefit from *moderate exercise* without endangering your health or your baby's growth. "Moderate," here means one hour of exercising three times a week.

For pregnant women, the American College of Obstetricians and Gynecologists recommends:

- Limiting a strenuous workout to 15 minutes.
- Keeping your heart rate under 140 beats a minute.
- Keeping your temperature under 100 degrees Fahrenheit.

You may certainly practice yoga techniques during pregnancy, or if you wish, find an exercise center or a local Y that has an exercise program designed especially for pregnant women.

## Stretching Exercises That Relieve Cramps

Here are a number of exercises that will help you relieve cramping and muscle strain during pregnancy:

*The Heel Stretch.* While lying on your back, point your heel away from your body, as shown in this illustration:

The heel stretch is effective in relieving cramps and sciatic pain.

*The Knee-to-Chest Stretch.* While lying on your back, slowly (a) bend and raise your right leg, (b) place both hands around your knee, and (c) pull the knee toward your chest. Repeat the process with the left knee. The knee-to-chest stretch effectively relieves leg cramps and sciatic pain.

*The One-Leg Stand.* When one leg feels cramped, stand tall and bend the knee of the *other* leg. By putting all your body weight on the cramped leg, you will reduce the cramping considerably.

*Shoulder and Arm Swings.* Slowly shrug your shoulders tightly and then stop. Now swing your arms in a circular fashion. The increased circulation will help relieve a tingling sensation or a feeling or numbness.

## Hydrotherapy

You may safely take warm or cool baths, but do *not* use a hot tub while you are pregnant. Avoid temperature extremes in any hydrotherapy techniques.

## Your Emotions and Your Health

Your emotions play a central role in your health during pregnancy. Be aware that from time to time you may experience special changes in your emotions, such as unexpected mood swings, impatience, irritability, resentment, or other negative feelings connected with your pregnancy. You may even have strange, perhaps frightening, dreams. Through it all, remember that such feelings and experiences are quite common and natural. Acknowledge these feelings—don't hide them.

## Handling Postpartum Depression

After childbirth, many women experience *postpartum depression*, a condition characterized by restlessness, fatigue, hypersensitivity, irritability, and ambivalence toward the newborn child.

Postpartum depression may last days, weeks, or months, and unfortunately, there is no known way to prevent this condition. However, as a result of their study of mothers at New Jersey's Englewood Hospital, Brenda Krause Eheart and Susan Karol Martel have a number of good suggestions that may help relieve postpartum depression:

- "Get plenty of rest and sleep.
- "Arrange in advance for baby-sitters.
- "Don't move to a new neighborhood just before or after the birth.
- "Worry less about how tidy the house is.
- "Get experienced help with the baby, if possible.
- "Have your husband do more at home and reduce outside activities somewhat, if possible.
- "Continue to socialize as a couple, but less often than before.
- "Continue your outside interests, but limit your outside responsibilities."

[Jane E. Brody, "Personal Health," *New York Times*, May 11, 1983, Section C, p. 6.]

## For Your Information

Many organizations across the country are excellent resources for pregnant women, new mothers, and their families. Here are some:

Ms. Barbara Feldman, Director
The Fertility Awareness Center
342 East 15 Street (#D)
New York, NY 10003
(212) 475-4490

Maternity Center Association
48 East 92 Street
New York, NY 10028
(212) 369-7300

Council of Guilds for Infant Survival
1800 M. Street, N.W.
Washington, DC 20036
(202) 833-2253

International Childbirth Education
  Association
P.O. Box 20852
Milwaukee, WI 53220

In the New York area, contact:

Ms. Marguerite Perenelli
587 Grelley Avenue
Staten Island, NY 10306
(718) 979-3552

NAPSAC Inc. (1)
P.O. Box 267
Marble Hill, MO 63764

ACHI (2)
P.O. Box 1219
Cerritos, CA 90701
(714) 994-5880

ASPO-NY (3)
P.O. Box 725, Midtown Station
New York, NY 10018

La Leche League International, Inc.
9616 Minneapolis Avenue
Franklin Park, IL 60131
(312) 455-7730

The American College of
  Nurse-Midwives
1012 14th Street, N.W.
Suite 801
Washington, DC 20005
(202) 347-5445

SHARE (4)
St. John's Hospital
800 East Carpenter
Springfield, IL 62769

(1) *NAPSAC* stands for National Association of Parents & Professionals for Safe Alternatives in Childbirth.

(2) *ACHI* stands for Association for Childbirth at Home International.

(3) *APSO* stands for American Society for Psychoprophylaxis in Obstetrics.

(4) A support group for parents who have suffered late miscarriages, stillbirths, and infant deaths.

# 36

## Respiratory Disorders

The human respiratory system is responsible for several essential functions, primarily:

- Supplying oxygen to every cell in the body.
- Removing body wastes.
- Providing the air needed for speech.
- Providing the air needed to filter and remove infectious agents.

Because the respiratory system performs such basic, important functions, respiratory problems can be rather serious, especially if they are misdiagnosed or left untreated.

### Common Respiratory Problems

The most common problems that affect the respiratory system are discussed next.

*Allergy-Induced Disorders.* Allergic bronchitis, asthma, allergic sinusitis, and hay fever are among the problems that can be induced by allergies.

*Chronic Bronchitis.* Think of chronic bronchitis as an inflammation of the airwaves. Characterized by spitting and coughing up mucus, chronic bronchitis continues for months and generally returns every year. Cigarette smoking is probably a major factor in most cases of chronic bronchitis, but other contributing factors may include fatigue, air pollution, and malnutrition.

If chronic bronchitis is left untreated, it can lead to emphysema, a far worse disorder.

*The Common Cold.* The common cold is an inflammation of the mucous membranes in the respiratory passages. We routinely lump many different disorders under the broad label "cold," but there are really several distinct types, named for the specific area in the upper-respiratory tract that is affected. *Rhinitis* is a cold centered in the nose; *pharyngitis* is a cold in the throat, and *laryngitis* is a cold in the voice box.

The cause of the common cold is still not clear. As many as 100 viruses have been identified as causing colds, but there are probably other contributing factors that combine with these viruses, including a low immune response, or contact with droplets expelled by an infectious person.

*Coughing.* Coughing is nature's way of cleaning out the respiratory system and raising mucus and phlegm. Because coughing is often natural and healthy, suppressing a cough is not always wise.

Only in the later stages of a respiratory infection—when a dry, hacking cough can disrupt sleep—is coughing not beneficial. for these dry, hacking coughs, try an herbal cough syrup. See page 171 for an effective recipe.

*Asthma.* Asthma, a condition often associated with children, affects many adults as well. Although asthma is seldom fatal, it is an exceptionally frightening, annoying condition marked by "attacks" during which the asthma sufferer has difficulty breathing. The length of an attack may vary from a few minutes to several days. Likewise, the severity of an attack will vary from one person to another and from one occurrence to another. In many cases, asthma may last a few years, then disappear.

During an asthma attack, certain specific things occur: The bronchial tubes become much smaller as a result of muscle spasms and swelling. Mucus clogs the small bronchial tubes. Stale air becomes trapped in the bronchial tubes. Afterward, breathing once again returns to normal, although the chest area may feel tender.

Technically speaking, asthma may really be a collection of symptoms, rather than one specific disorder, because many things may bring on asthma attacks. For example, asthma attacks may be brought on by:

| | |
|---|---|
| Allergies | Environmental chemicals |
| Food sensitivity | Common household products (such as air fresheners) |
| Weather changes | Dust |
| Certain exercises | Pollen in the air |
| Exertion | Pets |
| Paint | Strong emotions |

In addition, asthma can be caused by exposure to the toxic fumes released while meats and other foods are heat-sealed in plastic wrapping. Known as "meat-wrapper's asthma," this condition can be prevented by using alternatives to heat-sealing plastic; for example, ties or tapes.

*Emphysema.* Emphysema is marked by very heavy, very difficult breathing and abnormal swelling. In cases of emphysema, the lungs lose their elasticity and, as a result, can no longer hold open the air pathways. As the small air sacs in the lungs are destroyed, breathing becomes more and more difficult.

Cigarette smoking is certainly a major cause of emphysema, although other respiratory diseases and congenital factors may also be responsible in many cases.

*Influenza.* Commonly known as "the flu," influenza is a lower-respiratory infection. Although influenza sometimes appears to be no more than a very bad cold, it is potentially life-threatening to certain groups of people, for example, to heavy smokers and to people with severe asthma or heart disease.

The symptoms of influenza often include a high fever (as high as 106 degrees Fahrenheit) accompanied by chills, fatigue, joint and muscle pain, and headaches.

But many cases will also include additional symptoms, such as digestive problems, abdominal pain, diarrhea, vomiting, and hoarseness.

Children may also exhibit swollen glands and red, watery, itchy eyes.

*Pneumonia.* The primary causes of pneumonia, an inflammation of the small air sacs in the lungs, include allergies, viruses, fungal infections and inhalation of poisonous gases.

Symptoms will vary widely, but they typically include intestinal problems, coughing up phlegm streaked with blood, fever, chills, chest pain and muscular aches and pains.

*Pleurisy.* The membrane that encloses each lung and lines the chest cavity is known as the "pleura." *Pleurisy* describes an inflammation of this membrane.

The severity of pleurisy will vary from one case to another. In some instances, pleurisy can be temporary and rather harmless; in others, it can be dangerous and life-threatening.

## Foods to Avoid

In respiratory disorders, try to avoid the foods that many asthmatics are particularly sensitive to:

| | |
|---|---|
| Milk | Chocolate |
| Orange juice | Butter |
| Fish | Peanut butter |
| Nuts | |

## Effective Supplements

Many supplements can be especially helpful in avoiding and relieving respiratory disorders:

*Vitamin B₆.* In a Columbia University study, a daily dose of 100 milligrams of vitamin $B_6$ produced fewer and less-severe asthma attacks and at the same time reduced shortness of breath and other symptoms. But for best results, many nutritionists recommend taking 200 milligrams daily, especially for asthmatic children.

*Vitamin C.* Because vitamin C expands the air passages, it is especially effective in relieving the effects of colds and asthma symptoms. Furthermore, vitamin C has been found to reduce: The number of attacks in asthmatics. The number of attacks with severe symptoms. The severity of bronchospasms. [*Tropical and Geographical Medicine*, Vol. 32, No. 2, 1980, p. 00.]

*L-Cysteine.* This amino acid protects the body from many of the chemicals found in tobacco smoke and as a result of air pollution—chemicals that have been identified as factors in lung cancer and emphysema.

*Vitamin A.* Vitamin A reduces both the frequency and the severity of upper-respiratory infections.

*Zinc.* Zinc may actually attack and inactivate the virus that causes colds. Take two 23 milligram tablets of zinc every waking hour for one week. [*Medical World,* February 13, 1984.]

The benefits of zinc go beyond simply controlling cold symptoms. Studies showed that sucking on zinc lozenges (50 milligrams every two hours) reduced the recovery period to three or four days, instead of the usual seven days.

One possible minor side effect of zinc supplementation is a change in the sense of taste (a side effect that ends when supplementation ends). No other side effects have been reported.

## Juice Therapy

Use Juice Therapy Formula #5 (see Appendix) for relief from any respiratory disorder—especially asthma, bronchitis, pneumonia, and emphysema. Also valuable for respiratory disorders is a combination of celery juice and parsnip juice.

For emphysema, add four ounces of raw potato juice to Juice Therapy Formula #12 (page 214).

## The Most Effective Herbs

The herbs of choice for general respiratory disorders are:

| | |
|---|---|
| Yarrow flowers | Goldenseal |
| Skullcap | Echinacea |
| Boneset | Sarsaparilla |
| Elder flowers | Capsicum |
| Peppermint leaves | Thyme |
| Cinnamon bark | Eucalyptus |
| Peruvian bark | Wild cherry bark |
| Slippery elm bark | Red raspberry |

In addition, here are some specific herbal remedies for specific disorders:
*For Head Congestions:* Raw garlic.
*For Reducing Infection:* Goldenseal capsules.
*For Asthma:* These general herbs are effective for asthma:

| | |
|---|---|
| Cherry | Garlic |
| Onion | Rosemary |
| Horehound | Elecampane |
| Eucalyptus | Thyme |
| Lungwort | Mullein |
| Pleurisy root | |

A tea made from ephedra leaves is very effective for relieving asthmatic attacks. Ephedra is an old folk remedy. The commonly used drug ephedrine is derived from this herb.

Take stinging nettle tea for a couple of months.

*For Chest Congestion and Sore Lungs:* Eucalyptus.

*For Coughing with Phlegm:* Try cowslip, lungwort, eucalyptus leaf, peppermint leaf, pleurisy root, coltsfoot, mallow, and plantain.

Licorice is a very effective expectorant. If you wish, make your own licorice cough syrup: To 1 quart of distilled water, add one ounce each of licorice root, powdered slippery elm bark, flaxseed, and boneset. Simmer the mixture for 20 minutes. Strain the mixture, then add one pint of molasses. Take two tablespoons every hour.

NOTE: This cough syrup is an *expectorant*—that is, a remedy that *induces* coughing in an effort to dislodge the mucous secretions from the air passages. Remedies that *suppress* coughing, called "antitussives," temporarily calm the nervous system and do not induce coughing. Antitussives are not recommended.

*For Chronic Bronchitis:* Coltsfoot.

*For Head Colds:* Garlic, sage, and cayenne.

*For Chest Colds:* Try one of these popular herbal combinations for relief from chest colds: (1) Yarrow, elder flower, and peppermint; (2) Bayberry bark and ginger root; or (3) Boneset, elder, yarrow, and ginger.

*For Thick, Sticky Mucus:* Try one of these combinations:

1. Mix 2 parts coltsfoot, 1 part horehound, and 1 part licorice.
2. Combine sage, marshmellow root, coltsfoot, and comfrey.
3. Combine elecampane, white horehound, coltsfoot, and fennel.

*For Nasal Congestion:* Ephedra.

## Aroma Therapy: How Oils Act in Respiratory Conditions

Oils act in three very specific but very different ways that make them especially effective in treating respiratory disorders.

1. The *expectorant action* of an oil induces coughing up phlegm and mucus. The strongest oils for expectorant action are eucalyptus and lemon, which are most effective when used in steam inhalation.

2. The *antiseptic action* of an oil heals infections. The most effective healing oils for respiratory problems are essences of garlic and bergamot, for healing infections caused by the diphtheria bacillus; camphor oil, for pneumonia; eucalyptus oil, for influenza; and cinnamon, eucalyptus, and black pepper oils, for general respiratory infections.

You can take some of the healing oils orally. In addition, you can use them topically in a number of different ways: You can apply them in a friction chest rub. You can use them to massage along the spine, around the upper back and along the vertebrae in the neck area; or you can use them in compresses.

3. The *antispasmodic action* of an oil prevents muscle spasms. The most effective antispasmodic oils are clary, fennel, rose, and thyme.

Through these three specific actions, oils offer great relief from respiratory disorders.

## Aroma Therapy: Using Oils for Specific Disorders

Now let's see some of the ways in which oils can be used to treat specific respiratory disorders:

*For Asthma:* Virtually any essence that is generally helpful in respiratory disorders will be helpful in asthma conditions. Among the most popular oils are:

| | |
|---|---|
| Aniseed | Onion |
| Cajeput | Origanum |
| Garlic | Peppermint |
| Hyssop | Pine |
| Lavender | Rosemary |
| Lemon | Sage |
| Marjoram | Savory |
| Niaouli | Thyme |

*For Acute Bronchitis:* Oil of cajeput, eucalyptus, garlic, lavender, lemon, onion, pine, and savory.

*For Chronic Bronchitis:* All the essences listed for acute bronchitis are useful in chronic bronchitis. In addition, sandalwood and thyme are effective.

*For Coughs:* Place a few drops of essence of cypress on your pillow to control spasmodic coughs. Essences of aniseed, eucalyptus, and hyssop are also helpful.

*For Emphysema:* Essences of cypress, garlic, hyssop, and thyme.

*For Hiccups:* Place a few drops of essence of tarragon on your tongue.

*For Influenza:* Essences of cinnamon, clove, eucalyptus, lemon, naiouli, and thyme.

*For Pneumonia:* Essences of eucalyptus, lavender, lemon, niaouli, and pine.

*For Pleurisy:* Essence of onion.

*For Whooping Cough:* Essences of basil, cypress, garlic, lavender, niaouli, origanum, rosemary, terebinth, and thyme.

## Aroma Therapy: Getting the Most Out of Oils

To get the most out of the oils and the techniques described above, be sure to follow these guidelines:

• Combine no more than *four* oils in any one formula.

• When you do combine oils, add 7 drops of each essence. (For children's remedies, use only 3 drops of each essence.)

• Add the essences to a glass of warm water.

• Take the remedy three times a day, 10 minutes before each meal.

## Edgar Cayce Remedy

In his readings, Edgar Cayce recommended inhalant formulas for respiratory disorders. For an effective steam inhalant, mix these five ingredients: tincture benzoin, eucalyptus oil, turpentine oil, pine needle oil, and tincture tolu balsam.

## Visualization Exercise to Help You Breathe

A number of visualization techniques work very well in relieving respiratory disorders, especially emphysema and asthma, by reducing the amount of stress placed on the lungs. In addition, self-hypnosis is very effective for reducing both the frequency and the severity of asthma attacks.

Try this visualization technique to help you with any respiratory disorder:

Step 1. Find a quiet place where you will not be disturbed. Sit in a straight-back chair with both your feet flat on the floor and place your hands palms up on your knees.

Step 2. Close your eyes. Inhale and exhale long and slowly *into your lower abdomen, not into your chest alone.*

Step 3. As you inhale, visualize your bronchial tubes and lungs slowly expanding. With each cycle of inhaling and exhaling, you can *see* your bronchial tubes opening wider.

Step 4. Complete your visualization by (a) taking a long, deep breath, (b) slowly exhaling, and (c) gradually opening your eyes. Sit quietly for a few minutes as you become aware once again of your surroundings.

Step 5. Slowly begin to wiggle your fingers and toes. Rise only when you feel acclimated to your surroundings.

## Acupressure and Massage

To relieve asthma, place pressure on the floor of the mouth, especially near the foot of the tone.

Also, try lymphatic kneading.

## Exercise

If you suffer from any respiratory disorder, build up your abdominal muscles to make breathing easier. Also, take long, slow walks to build up your endurance and your strength.

In addition to these general suggestions, here are some specific recommendations for exercises that are especially effective for specific conditions:

*For Asthma.* If you have asthma, do not exercise when you are feeling any attack symptoms because exercise may aggravate your condition. In all other cases, be sure to break up your exercise program into short intervals. In other words, don't overdo it! [*Annals of Allergy*, February 1982.]

*For Emphysema and Bronchitis:* Studies show that daily exercising on a stationary cycle may stop the negative progression of emphysema and bronchitis and also improve these conditions.

## Hydrotherapy

Hydrotherapy is very useful for relieving respiratory conditions.

*For Coughs.* To break up a cough, apply a cold compress to your chest in the evening before going to bed. Moist compresses increase circulation and remove impurities through the skin. Prepare the compress as follows:

Dip a towel or a facecloth made from cotton (or any other natural fiber) in very cold water—water to which you've added a few ice cubes. Wring out the towel so that it is still moist, not dripping wet. Fold the towel twice to create four layers, then place the towel on your chest. Make sure that you are not near a drafty area.

Now fold a second towel, a dry towel, and use it to cover the wet compress. When folded, the dry towel should be large enough to cover the underlying wet compress. If you wish, place a rubber sheet under the wet compress so that no water drips onto your bed.

Wait about 10 minutes. Then dip the cloth in the cold water once again and apply it to the chest area. As before, be sure to cover this wet towel with a dry towel. Every 15 minutes, repeat the process of rewetting the towel. After 1 hour, remove the cold compress, dry the chest area, and cover yourself quickly.

Afterward, place the cloth in boiling water. Do not reuse the cloth until it has been cleaned in boiling water.

Another remedy to break up a cough is to add thyme to a hot bath and soak for a while.

*For Mucus.* Take a high-pressure cold-water shower, letting the water hit the chest area especially. Also, bend over and let the high-pressure stream of water hit your upper back.

*For Lung Disorders.* Use thyme or pine needle essences, both of which have an antiseptic effect, help thin mucus, and act as expectorants.

## Homeopathy

A number of homeopathic remedies are effective for respiratory disorders:

### For Chest Colds:
- *With Mucus:* Salix nig.
- *Accompanied by a Dry Cough, Sore Chest, and Mucus:* Gelsenium.
- *With Short Dry Cough:* Coffea.
- *With Soreness and Mucus:* Eupatorium perf.

### For Coughs:
- *General Coughs:* Aconite and hepar sulph.
- *With Hoarseness and Dry Throat:* Bryonia and spongia.
- *With Laryngitis:* Causticum.
- *With Raw Sore Throat:* Populus can.

### For Head Colds:
- *With Runny Nose and Swollen Sinuses:* Sanguinaria can.
- *With Runny Nose:* Pulsatilla and hydrastis.
- *With Watery, Burning Eyes:* Arsenicum.
- *With Heavy Congestion:* Aconite.

### For Runny Nose and Sinus Congestion:
- Euphrasia.

## Tissue Salts

Note how tissue salts can be used for specific respiratory conditions:

*For General Respiratory Problems*: Calcium phosphate.

*For Bronchial Asthma:* Calcium phosphate. When bronchial asthma is accompanied by a thick yellow expectoration, use potassium sulfate.

*For Asthma:* Sodium sulfate, especially when the asthma is accompanied by a thick green mucus.

*For Congestion:* Phosphate of iron 6X.

*For Hard, Dry Cough With Fever and Soreness:* Phosphate of iron 6X.

*To Reduce Mucus:* Potassium chloride. (This is to reduce, specifically, a white mucus on the tongue, as well as any other secretions associated with bronchitis, colds, coughs, and runny noses.)

*For Acute Rhinitis, Colds, and Coughs:* Phosphate of iron, potassium chloride, and sodium chloride in combination.

*For Anyone Especially Susceptible to Colds:* Phosphate or iron, potassium chloride, and sodium chloride in combination.

*For Sore Throats:* Phosphate of iron, potassium chloride, and potassium phosphate in combination.

*For Winter Coughs, Colds, Etc.:* Phosphate of iron, potassium chloride, and sodium chloride in combination.

*For Fever and Yellow, Slimy Expectoration:* Phosphate of iron and potassium sulfate.

## Weather Changes

Changes in the weather affect respiratory conditions in certain ways. For example, *bronchial asthma* will be aggravated by very cool air, great heat, cold air from the northwest, or high humidity. *Bronchitis* will be aggravated on foggy days.

## Also of Interest

The following information related to respiratory conditions may be helpful to you.

• Here are two good tips that will be sure to help *any* respiratory condition: Drink plenty of fluids and get proper rest.

• Substances that are known to aggravate children's asthma symptoms are aspirin, tartrazine, an artificial coloring agent, certain artificial flavorings, and monosodium glutamate (MSG). Children who have eaten foods with MSG may not show symptoms until 12 hours later, in some cases. [*Medical Journal of Australia*, November 28, 1981.]

• When you take *oral* steroid medications for asthma (or for any other condition, for that matter), your adrenal gland stops producing cortisone. If you plan to reduce or completely discontinue taking the steroid medications, you *must* be sure to do so *gradually*, and only under the supervision of a competent medical professional. Otherwise, you may create a cortisone deficiency in your body.

• Biofeedback is essentially a sophisticated form of relaxation training. Because asthma involves muscular spasms, biofeedback may be very helpful in asthma conditions.

• Here are some ways in which you can reduce fevers:

1. Take ginger baths in a bathtub with the curtains closed. While sitting in the tub, drink ginger teas with lemon and a pinch of cayenne pepper. Keep a cool pack at the back of your neck while you are in the bath.

2. Soak your feet in warm water.

3. Take a warm-water enema.

4. Supplement with Superacidophilus or Megadophilus brands of acidophilus.

• Music therapy—more specifically, playing wind instruments—has been used successfully to treat children with various respiratory disorders, especially asthma.

• Negative ion therapy is extremely beneficial in healing respiratory tissues, particularly in cases of respiratory tract allergies such as allergic bronchitis, asthma, allergic sinusitis, and hay fever.

• "Passive smoking," the effects of others' smoking, can affect your respiratory condition. For example, if you have asthma, living in the same house with a smoker increases your risk of attack.

## Alex J.'s Annual Cold

Alex J. eats well, and he exercises regularly. However, he has a great deal of emotional stress, and he has various allergic nose and throat disorders that weaken his immunity to colds. Thus every winter, when he comes in contact with someone who has a cold, he, too, invariably catches it.

And not a *minor* cold! Whenever Alex catches a cold, he has a rough hacking cough at night, constant congestion all day, and a runny nose that alternates with a stuffed-up nose. Worse, his symptoms always last a full two weeks.

Then one day, Alex began following a specific program for preventing and treating colds:

1. At the first sign of a cold, Alex got two or three days of bed rest and followed a proper diet. He increased his intake of warm fluids to maintain body fluids and loosen mucus.

2. Alex avoided stress.

3. He used steam with essence of eucalyptus or essence of thyme to expectorate mucus; and he lubricated his nostrils with a comfrey salve to reduce irritation.

4. To reduce pain, inflammation, and fever, Alex used white willow bark tablets, which contain salicin, a natural substance that is related to aspirin.

5. He supplemented with vitamins A and C.

6. Alex eliminated immune-depressing stimulants such as alcohol, tobacco, coffee, tea, chocolate, and sugar.

7. To prevent cracking of his nasal mucus membranes, he used a humidifier to offset the effects of the heat in his apartment.

8. Alex began using herbal teas and following juice therapy formulas with plenty of carrot and citrus juices. He also went through a general internal detoxification program.

9. As his symptoms changed, Alex used whichever homeopathic remedies were appropriate.

Following this program, Alex can now effectively stop the full symptoms of a cold from setting in by following a natural healing approach. Now his "colds" typically last for only a day or two—rarely more than three days—as compared with the 14-day colds he once had.

# 37

# Sinusitis

In the front of your skull are four pairs of sinus cavities that supply mucus to the nose. An inflammation of one or more of these sinus passages, usually the *nasal* sinuses, is called "sinusitis." The inflammation may be caused by poor dental hygiene or mouth hygiene, tonsillitis, a cold, or a sore throat.

The symptoms of sinusitis may include:

| | |
|---|---|
| Fatigue | Coughing |
| Headaches | Nasal congestion |
| Pain around the eyes | Mucous discharge |
| Light fever | Increased susceptibility to infection |

The pain, which results because the cavity is blocked, may be extreme and may be accompanied by fever and pus.

The treatment for sinusitis centers around opening the blocked passageway by vapor inhalation techniques, by reducing the fever, and by bed rest.

## Your Supplementation Program

Because sinus problems often result from a vitamin A deficiency, be sure to include vitamin A in your daily supplementation.

Here is an effective daily program:

| | |
|---|---|
| Vitamin A | Phosphorus |
| Vitamin C | Calcium |
| Vitamin D | Zinc |
| Vitamin E | |

## Herbs that Relieve Sinusitis

Two herbs that can help you relieve sinusitis are sage and slippery elm bark.

## Aroma Therapy

Use these essences: eucalyptus, lavender, lemon, niaouli, peppermint, mint, and thyme.

## Juice Therapy

For mucus congestion, try Juice Therapy Formula #5, and one hour later follow it up by drinking a combination of 12 ounces of carrot juice and 4 ounces of radish juice.

Horseradish, one of the ingredients in Formula #5, dissolves mucus. The radish juice then cleanses the body of this dissolved mucus, according to N. W. Walker, the pioneer of juice therapy.

## Hydrotherapy

Try these three hydrotherapy techniques to open up your sinus passages and relieve the symptoms of sinusitis:

1. Two or three times a day, drape a hot towel over your face for an hour or more. If you prefer, you may use a heating pad or a hot water bottle instead.

2. Sit in a steaming-hot tub.

3. Use a humidifier to moisturize the air in your home and prevent excessive drying of your nasal membranes.

# 38

# Skin Disorders

Your skin, the largest organ of your body, has three primary functions:

- To protect your body.
- To help eliminate waste matter.
- To control your body temperature.

Skin problems can result from any number of causes, both physical or emotional. For example, all of the following can affect your skin: fluoridated water, birth control pills, perspiration, heat, humidity, and other environmental factors. Thus natural healers do not regard skin disorders in isolation; instead, they view skin problems as part of the total system.

## Common Skin Problems

The most common skin problems are described below.

*Acne.* The cause of acne—inflammations and irritations of the skin—is unknown, but many contributing factors *are* known, including these:

*Heredity.* Children whose parents had acne have a greater chance of getting acne, even if only *one* parent had acne.

*Oily Skin.* Oily hair and oily skin, characterized by an overabundance of sebum, the fatty substance produced by the sebaceous glands, contribute to acne.

*Androgen Levels.* Male sex hormones, androgens, regulate both the size and the activity of oil-producing glands.

*Foods.* Rich, oily foods, such as chocolate and fried foods, contribute to acne.

*Heat and Humidity.* Heat and humidity may aggravate an already-existing condition by swelling the pores and the canal through which oil travels, thereby blocking the canal and causing what is known as "tropical acne."

*Friction and Sweating.* Sweating and friction may combine to cause acne. For example, (1) if you wear a headband while playing tennis, you may develop acne on your forehead; (2) if you play football, you may develop acne where your shoulder pads rub your skin.

*Menstruation.* Teenage girls are especially susceptible to what is known as "menstrual acne."

*Acrodermatitis Enteropathica.* This rare skin condition, caused by a disorder in zinc metabolism, is inherited. The condition is characterized by:

- Skin lesions that do not heal.
- Stunted growth.
- Poor nutrient absorption.
- Disrupted bowel function.

Acrodermatitis enteropathica appears early in life, but it is never found in children while they are being breast-fed, although it may arise after they are weaned. Interestingly, however, the symptoms once again disappear if a weaned child returns to breast-feeding. Perhaps the zinc that the child ingests through breast-feeding is more easily metabolized than the zinc in cow's milk or in formula.

Although no cure is yet known, acrodermatitis enteropathica can be controlled through nutritional therapies that will leave the child symptom-free.

*Bedsores.* Bedsores, a form of ulcers, appear on the skin when the flow of body fluids is disrupted to that area. Often, bedsores begin when part of the body is subjected to tremendous pressure or friction. Bedsores are common in bedridden people, for example, people who are hospitalized or institutionalized for long periods of time.

Most susceptible are the elderly, people who have poor personal hygiene habits, and individuals who suffer from malnutrition or preexisting infections.

Moisture and heat contribute to bedsores and will aggravate an existing condition. If left untreated, bedsores can become gangrenous and may be life-threatening.

*Boils.* A boil is an infected, pus-filled nodule on the skin. Natural healers consider boils the body's natural way of eliminating internal toxins and impurities, necessitated by low resistance and poor nutrition.

*Burns.* A burn is an injury to tissue caused by chemicals, electricity, heat, or radiation. As a result of the destruction of tissues, the skin area has undergone a great loss of body fluids, nitrogen, and a number of nutrients, primarily sodium and potassium.

*Chapped Lips.* If you have chapped lips only when you awake, then perhaps you are breathing through your mouth while you sleep. Use one of the vitamin lip balms or colorless lip balms available in health food stores. Use it before you go to bed, if you often wake up with chapped lips.

*Dandruff.* Dandruff is a mild form of seborrheic dermatitis on the scalp. See "Dermatitis."

*Dermatitis.* There are a number of different kinds of dermatitis. Two of the most common, *dry skin* and *seborrhea,* are discussed as follows.

*Dry Skin.* To treat dry skin, help the skin to self-correct the condition through (1) careful washing and (2) by increasing skin circulation. In the evening use a gentle nonabrasive cleanser and a lotion free of "synthetic" oils such as mineral oil. Treatments that recommend covering the skin with oils, lotions, and creams will bring only temporary relief. Worse, they may make the skin dependent on these applications and decrease the skin's ability to manufacture its own protective oils.

*Seborrheic Dermatitis.* This condition is characterized by extreme scaling of the skin; so extreme that it may resemble a very heavy, wild case of dandruff. The scaling may be noticed behind the ears, on the nose, around the eyebrows, in the genital areas, under the arms, and in every other imaginable crease or skin fold. The scales may be accompanied by oozing, crusting, and extreme redness.

The cause of seborrheic dermatitis is not known, but it is aggravated by physical and emotional stress. It is commonly found in people suffering from neurological disorders.

*Eczema.* Many skin disorders can properly be labeled "eczema," but all exhibit a unique pattern of similar symptoms:

First, the skin becomes red and swollen. Next, the skin beings to blister and ooze. Then, in the final stage, the skin becomes scabbed and crusted. If the condition becomes chronic, the skin will then peel, chafe, thicken, and change color.

The causes of eczema include infections, irritations, genetic predisposition, reactions to drugs, poor circulation, reactions to toxic substances, allergies, and a drying effect that results from low humidity and cold weather.

*Itching.* Literally *hundreds* of factors, both environmental and emotional, can cause itching. If itching accompanies a skin rash, finding the cause may be somewhat simpler, but itching often appears and disappears for no apparent reasons.

Itching may be caused by kidney, liver, or thyroid disease, cancer, very dry skin (especially in the elderly) in wintertime and in very humid weather, allergic reactions, or food sensitivity.

*Psoriasis.* Psoriasis is a noncontagious, recurring disorder characterized by red circular patches of skin covered with dry, silvery scales. The patches may get larger.

Psoriasis is most often found on the arms, legs, lower back, scalp, and ears. Heredity may be a factor in this condition.

*Shingles.* Viral infection causing painful blisters.

*Warts.* Warts are skin tumors caused by viral infections.

## Good Nutrition: What to Avoid in Your Diet

To follow a nutrition program that will help promote healthy skin and treat any skin disorders, be sure to avoid:

| | | |
|---|---|---|
| Yeast | Alcohol | Strong spices |
| Wheat products | Black teas | Very hot foods and beverages |
| Refined sugar | Coffee | Cow's milk |

Cow's milk is a common allergen for people with skin problems. Although not every one with a skin problem is allergic to cow's milk, many people who replace cow's milk with goat's milk or soy milk get rid of their rashes or dermatitis symptoms.

## Good Nutrition: What to Include in Your Diet

Be sure to include essential fatty acids in your diet. Studies show that EFAs are a major factor in skin disorders. To obtain EFAs, add a few tablespoons of sesame oil, safflower oil, or sunflower oil daily, either to your salad or to the foods you cook. Other good sources of EFAs are raw, unsalted nuts and seeds.

## Good Nutrition: How to Treat Specific Skin Conditions

Here are some specific recommendations for different kinds of skin disorders.

*For Acne:* Some food allergies may contribute to acne, especially allergies to dairy products and wheat. See "Allergies" on page 12.

Natural healers dispute dermatologists' claims that foods do not aggravate acne conditions. The reason is simply that many severe acne conditions *do* clear up if you avoid certain foods such as chocolate, coffee, cola beverages, fried foods, nuts, especially dry-roasted nuts, and whole-milk products.

*For Burns:* Healing burned tissue requires lots of time and a specialized nutrition program that may require intravenous feeding.

If you are an average-size person, increase your caloric intake to 5,000 or 6,000 calories a day and your protein intake to 200 grams a day. Also, eat many small meals rather than few large meals.

*For Bedsores:* A protein deficiency can contribute to or aggravate bedsores or ulcers. If your protein intake is not adequate, supplement your diet.

*For Eczema:* Protein deficiencies have also been found to cause eczema.

*For Psoriasis:* The cause of psoriasis is not known, but many patients see improvement in their conditions when they start a gluten-free diet and eliminate acidic foods, such as coffee, pineapples, tomatoes, soda, corn, nuts, and milk. [*Western Journal of Medicine,* November 1980.] An increased intake of animal protein may aggravate psoriasis.

## Supplements That Help

Many supplements are beneficial in treating skin disorders, including vitamins A, D, and C and zinc. Besides these general recommendations, note these suggestions for specific conditions:

*For Acne:* Zinc supplementation is highly recommended in acne cases. [*Nutrition Reviews,* February 1981.] But for many people with acne and other skin problems, the body may not be producing enough hydrochloric acid to fully utilize the zinc and other minerals in their diets, even though their intake of these minerals may be perfectly normal. As a result, even zinc and vitamin $B_{12}$ supplementation may not bring about the expected results.

To increase mineral absorption and improve digestion, supplementation with betaine hydrochloride or glutamic acid may be necessary. A physician can test for low hydrochloric acid production.

*For Acrodermatitis Enteropathica:* Under a physician's direction, take a *total* dosage of 150 milligrams of zinc each day. Your physician will help you divide this total into smaller doses.

*For Eczema:* Acidophilus is very beneficial for treating intractable eczema, as well as a wide range of other skin problems. [Sandler, "Lactobacillus for Vulvovaginitis," *The Lancet,* October 13, 1979, p. 791.]

*For Menstrual Acne:* Take vitamin $B_6$.

*For Bedsores:* take all nutrients that help heal wounds:

| | | |
|---|---|---|
| Vitamin A | Folic Acid | Vitamin C |
| Vitamin $B_2$ | Zinc | Riboflavin |
| Vitamin E | Vitamin B complex | Copper |

*For Boils:* Take vitamins C and E and zinc.

*For Burns:* For serious burns, supplementation is essential to healing. Minimum supplementation should include:

| | | |
|---|---|---|
| Vitamin C (2,000 mg) | Vitamin D | PABA |
| Thiamine (50 mg) | Vitamin $B_1$ | EFAs |
| Riboflavin (50 mg) | Vitamin $B_2$ | Potassium |
| Niacinamide (500 mg) | Vitamin $B_{12}$ | Zinc |
| Vitamin A | Vitamin E | Arginine |

*For Bruising and Inflammation:* Take the following supplements:

| | |
|---|---|
| Bioflavonoids (200 mg) | Bromelain (50 mg) |
| Vitamin C (200 mg) | Papain (50 mg) |
| Pantothenic Acid (200 mg) | Rutin (100 mg) |
| Zinc (amino acid chelate—20 mg) | |

*For Dandruff:* The best supplements for dandruff conditions are zinc, EFAs, vitamin $B_6$, vitamin E, and the B complex vitamins.

*For Dermatitis:* A deficiency in any of the B vitamins can cause dermatitis. Infants on fat-free diets who had dermatitis were cured with supplements of linoleic acid and vitamin $B_6$. [Jonathan V. Wright, *Dr. Wright's Book of Nutritional Therapy,* Emmaus, Pennsylvania, Rodale Press, 1979, p. 41.] Also, green barley juice (Green Magma brand) is very effective in relieving dermatitis symptoms.

People suffering from dermatitis often have white spots on their nails, indications of a zinc deficiency. Zinc supplementation may not show results for as long as two months, but more important, zinc can be toxic if supplemented for too long a time or in excessive doses. Therefore, contact a health professional before you experiment with zinc supplementation.

*For Dry, Rough, Flaking Skin:* Use vitamin A and EFAs.

*For Eczema:* Take six capsules of evening primrose oil twice a day. [*The Lancet,* November 20, 1982.] Also helpful is Green Magma, a brand name for the juice of young green barley plants. ["Therapeutic Experiment of the Young Green Barley Juice for the Treatment of Skin Diseases in the Main," *New Drugs and Clinical Application,* Vol. 26, No. 5, May 10, 1977.]

*For Hives:* Try a combination of zinc, vitamin C, and pantothenic acid.

*For Prickly Heat:* Even extreme cases of prickly heat will be helped by 1,000 milligrams of vitamin C each day.

*For Psoriasis:* Take niacin to heal the lesions caused by psoriasis. [*Skin and Allergy News,* July 1979.]

*For Sunburn:* Use vitamin E, both orally and topically.

## Amino Acid Therapy

Proline helps promote skin flexibility and is therefore useful for aging skin and for skin exposed to the sun.

## Juice Therapy

As a general therapy for any skin disorders, you may try Juice Therapy Formula #3. See the Appendix.

Unless you have arthritis, try this combination: mix green pepper juice and raw potato juice half-and-half.

Drink 16 ounces of carrot juice each day.

In addition, here are some juice therapies for specific conditions:

- For Boils: Try Juice Therapy Formulas #14, #17, and #20.
- For Acne: Mix the juice of carrots, lettuce, and spinach in equal parts.

## Herbal Remedies for Skin Disorders

General herbs that are useful for skin conditions include:

| White Oak Bark | Yellow Dock |
|---|---|
| Chaparral | Comfrey |
| Burdock | Periwinkle |

Specific herbal remedies include:

*For Acne and Dry Skin:* Jojoba oil.

*For Boils:* Flaxseed poultices are very effective topical remedies. Also, for internal cleansing, drink any of these teas:barberry, echinacea, goldenseal, burdock, cayenne, yellow dock.

*For Insect Bites and Stings:* Use an aloe gel poultice.

*For Poison Ivy and Poison Oak:* Spread aloe gel liberally over the affected area.

*For Shingles:* Rub the gel from the leaves of a fresh aloe plant onto the affected skin to soothe the pain.

*For Cuts, Scratches, and Splinters:* Spread aloe gel on the affected area. Also, make your own antiseptic, as described next.

## Make Your Own Herbal Antiseptic

Thyme and sage are two of the most powerful herbal antiseptics. You can make your own antiseptic with these herbs, as follows:

Fill a glass jar loosely with equal parts of sage and thyme. Fill the jar with vodka, cap the jar tightly, and let the mixture stand in a dark place for two weeks. After two weeks, strain the mixture.

Use this antiseptic to wash cuts or scratches. For infections, you may use this mixture to ash the area, then follow up with a commercial antiseptic, which will have a stronger effect.

## Aroma Therapy

Try these aroma therapy techniques:

*For Acne:* Essences of cajeput, juniper, and lavender.

*For Boils:* Essences of chamomile, lemon, onion, and thyme.

*For Burns:* Essences of chamomile, eucalyptus, geranium, lavender, niaouli, onion, rosemary, and sage.

*For Eczema:* Essence of citral ointment and the oils of chamomile, hyssop, and sage.

*For Psoriasis:* Essence of cajeput.

## Herbal Facial Steaming

Herbal facial steaming is a hyydrotherapy technique that helps open and clean pores, cleanses the skin, and reduces the action of the oil-producing glands. To get the most out of this effective technique, make a tea as follows:

1. Into a bowl place one heaping tablespoon of each of the herbs listed here (choose whichever formula is appropriate):

*Formula for Oily Skin:* Licorice root, rosebuds, and lemongrass.

*Formula for Acne and Blemished Skin:* Red clover, strawberry leaves, and lavender.

*Formula for Combination Skin* (that is, skin that is both dry and oily): Lavender, peppermint, licorice root, and chamomile.

2. Add two cups of boiling water. Cover the bowl with a tight lid, and let the tea steep for three to five minutes.

3. Remove the lid. Now position your head directly over the bowl and cover your head with a towel so that you can form a "tent" of sorts. For best results, tuck the ends of the towel under the bowl to create your own miniature steam cabinet.

4. Inhale the herbal steam. At the same time, the antiseptic oils will kill the germs responsible for your skin condition.

5. After five to ten minutes of steaming, wash your face with cool water.

[Kathi Keville, "Winter Complexion Care," *Vegetarian Times,* February, 1983, p. 51.]

## Other Hydrotherapy Techniques

In addition to facial steaming, try these hydrotherapy techniques:

*For Boils:* (1) Us hot compresses to relieve pain and increase healing. (2) Use a high-pressure cold-water spray. (3) Use a fenugreek seed plaster.

*For Itching:* Try an ice massage and cool packs to reduce itching. Avoid hot baths, which may increase itching.

*For General Skin Problems:* Try cool or tepid colloidal baths using one or a combination of the following: colloidal oatmeal, skim milk, powdered milk, cornstarch, baking soda.

[Emrika Paduṣ, *The Women's Encyclopedia of Natural Health and Healing,* Emmaus, Pennsylvania, Rodale Press, 1981, p. 457.

## Homeopathy

*For Acne:* Bromum. hepar. sulf., ledum pal, kali bromatum.

*For Shingles:* Mezereum.

*For Teenage Acne:* Kali bromatum is especially helpful for teenagers who have itchy skin, are having trouble sleeping, and are having unpleasant dreams. Sulfur is useful when the acne is chronic and the skin is rough and hard and is aggravated by washing.

*For Poison Oak and Poison Ivy:* Rhus. tox 3X, Crot. tig. 6X, anacardium 6X.

## Tissue Salts

*For General Skin Problems:* Alternate using calcium sulfate and calcium phosphate.

*For Acne, Scaling, Eczema, and Scalp Eruptions:* Potassium chloride, potassium sulfate, calcium sulfate, and silicic oxide.

*For Boils and Deep-Seated Pus Formations:* Silicea 6X.

*For Abscesses and Boils:* Calcium sulfate 6X.

## General Skin Care Techniques

Try to follow these general skin care suggestions:

1. Wear clothing and use bedsheets and towels made of 100 percent cotton or some other natural fiber.

2. When washing clothes, avoid fabric softeners and harsh detergents.

3. Avoid using soaps, especially if you have sensitive skin. Even soaps with aloe, cucumber, avocado, or other plant substances may be too harsh for very sensitive skin. Instead, use cleansing creams to remove dirt.

If you shower daily, use soap only on odor-producing parts of your body.

4. Use products that do *not* include coal tar or synthetic ingredients and preservatives. Read labels carefully: Most commercial skin care and cosmetic preparations *do* contain these ingredients.

The products that are most respected by skin care specialists are those manufactured by this company:

Dr. Hauschka Cosmetics Inc.
Route 138
Wyoming, RI 02898

## Special Skin Care Techniques

Try the following skin care techniques:

• Make a facial compress from grated cucumbers. Leave the compress on for one-half hour, then wash your face.

• Make a brewer's yeast facial mask: Cleanse your skin with a mixture of water and apple cider vinegar. Mix one teaspoon brewer's yeast with enough yogurt to form a thin paste. Apply this paste to your skin by patting the paste onto your face. Allow the paste to dry for 15 minutes. Rinse your face with warm water and then cold water. Blot your face dry.

• Steam your face once a week (unless steaming specifically aggravates your skin).

• Use a skin cream that contains vitamin $B_6$, which is very helpful in many different skin disorders.

## Other Therapies

Here are additional therapies that you may find useful in treating certain skin disorders.

*Acne.* The main treatment for mild acne is cleansing the skin two or three times a day with a nonsoap cleanser to remove excess oil. Be careful not to scrub too hard, especially in the summer when your skin may appear oilier. Excessive scrubbing only aggravates the condition.

Ultraviolet light and sunlight may help clear up some mild forms of acne. But if you are taking medication for acne, be sure to check with your doctor before you go in the sun. Direct sunlight may cause negative reactions if you are taking certain acne drugs.

*Athlete's Foot.* Try Athafut Lotion, a commercial product that is reported to be very effective. Athafut Lotion is available from:

General Research Laboratories, Inc.
139 Illinois Avenue
El Segundo, CA 90245

*Bedsores.* To prevent and treat bedsores, try these general measures:

1. Turn a bedridden person every two hours to relieve the constant pressure on one spot.

2. Avoid raising her or his head more than 30 degrees off the bed to reduce pressure at the bottom and the top of the spine.

3. Place loose clothing on a bedridden person to allow him or her greater movement and less restriction. Also, be sure that bedsheets and blankets are not too tight and do not restrict movement.

4. When you help a bedridden person to move, try to lift *up*, rather than pull the person *across* the bed. A pulling action causes skin friction and aggravates bedsores.

Here is more information related to bedsores:

Products that help reduce pressure and friction include air-filled mattresses, water beds, and special cushions and pads. But these products seldom do enough to effect any great improvement.

A special cushion sold under the brand name ''Sof-Care'' has produced very positive results. For more information, contact:

Marketing Department
Gaymar Industries
10 Centre Drive
Orchard Park, NY 14127

Sprinkle karaya, an enzyme vegetable gum, on an open wound and cover it with a plastic wrap similar to Saran and other commercial food wraps. In a hospital test, using karaya in this way helped ulcers to heal in only 7 to 14 days, depending on the severity of the bedsore.

Packing honey or sugar onto bedsores may also promote healing. Concentrated sugar and honey are known to have an antibacterial effect when applied topically. Lecithin has also been used topically to help treat bedsores.

Another remedy for bedsores is vitamin A and D ointment combined with zinc oxide cream and vitamin E oil. This mixture has been very successful. Of course, you may use Vitamin E by itself on bedsores.

*Boils.* Wash the infected area several times a day with an herbal antiseptic (see page 000). After each wash, apply vitamin A ointment.

*Burns.* Immediately after a burn, do *not* use any butter, grease, or ointments of any kind. Instead, plunge the burned area into ice water or wrap the area in a towel that has been soaked in ice water. This process will lessen the pain and the degree of blistering. At the same time, it will support healing.

Note these additional suggestions concerning burns:

The skin loses its natural lubrication as the result of a burn. To prevent scaling and flaking, apply cocoa butter, comfrey, or some other herbal moisturizer, a vitamin E ointment—even Crisco or a similar shortening—once or twice a day. [*Postgraduate Medicine*, May 1981.]

For eye burns caused by acids, alkalis, or other chemicals, flood the eye immediately with water and continue doing so repeatedly for 15 minutes. Then call an eye doctor or go to the emergency room of the nearest hospital to prevent further damage. Do so as quickly as possible.

Topical remedies used to spur healing as a result of burns include:

Aloe gel, which has antimicrobial and analgesic properties.

Spraying catalyst-altered water on the burn.

Soaking the burn in cold water.

Applying honey under a dry dressing every two or three days

Applying yogurt to the burn two or three times a day.

Using comfrey salve.

Applying chlorophyll.

*Dandruff.* Wash your hair with very mild, unmedicated soap. Rub a small amount of vitamin E oil into your scalp. Be sure to use only a small amount of the vitamin E oil or your hair will look greasy.

*Eczema (Dermatitis).* You have a number of options for avoiding and treating eczema:

1. Drink the juice of young green barley plants (Green Magma brand is available in health food stores). A protein in this juice has a strong anti-inflammatory action that relieves dermatitis.

2. After bathing, always apply an emollient cream.

3. Avoid climates with extreme changes of temperature. Very humid climates will aggravate the condition, while warm, dry climates seem to promote healing.

4. Avoid clothing made of synthetic and non-absorbent materials. Cotton is usually the best choice. Silk and wool can be rather irritating.

5. Use very mild laundry products, and be sure to rinse all clothes well.

6. Consider carefully whether any emotional factors can be contributing to your condition.

7. If you have dermatitis on your hands and must do wet work, wear cotton gloves under a pair of rubber gloves. The cotton gloves will both protect the inflamed hands and absorb sweat, which might aggravate the condition.

8. Cover the affected area with cotton gauze to reduce scratching throughout the day.

9. Avoid harsh soaps to reduce irritation. Use any baby soap that does not contain perfume, sulfur, or tar.

10. Avoid skin contact with any harsh chemicals—solvents, cleaning products, stain removers, and so on.

11. Do not squeeze or peel citrus fruits with your bare hands.

*Hives.* Many people who suffer from hives are really reacting to a sensitivity to certain foods, food additives, or chemical agents. If you are among these people, avoid substances such as tartrazine (the food coloring FD & C Yellow #5), BHT, BHA, carotene, nitrates, aspirin and salicylates (aspirin-like substances), benzoate preservatives, and penicillin

Physical stimuli, too, can cause hives: sunlight, heat, or cold. [*The Lancet*, November 3, 1979.]

*Itching.* Dab apple cider vinegar on the affected area.

*Psoriasis.* Remedies which are effective for psoriasis include hot baths, which provide relief in many cases.

Using ultrasound to raise the skin temperature to 110 degrees Fahrenheit for 30 minutes at a time has produced impressive results. This treatment requires two or three treatments a week for a few weeks. [*Archives of Dermatology*, August, 1980.]

Using vitamin E ointment to heal lesions is also an effective treatment for psoriasis.

*Sunburn.* Several remedies are effective in treating sunburn:

1. Apply aloe vera gel topically—it's very soothing.

2. Prepare calundula (marigold) vinegar, a classic sunburn remedy. Proceed as follows: Fill a jar with fresh marigold flowers. Then fill it with apple cider vinegar. Let the mixture stand for about two weeks, then strain the leaves.

Now, to make the sunburn formula, mix aloe vera juice with the vinegar in a 2:1 proportion. To speed up its healing effect, add vitamin E to this mixture.

3. Spray burns with catalyst-altered water. Splash and rub vinegar lightly onto the burn to reduce the sting and increase healing.

*Minor Skin Injuries.* For cuts, scrapes, scratches, insect bites, bruises, and some rashes, spray catalyst-altered water on the injury for quick relief.

*Sweat-Induced Skin Problems.* To prevent and treat sweat-induced skin problems:

• Wear loose clothing made from natural fibers.

• After exercising, remove sweaty clothing immediately and take a cool shower.

• Sprinkle cornstarch on your skin to prevent friction with your clothing, or use a combination of cornstarch and slippery elm bark. Reapply the cornstarch as necessary. Men, especially, should follow this procedure to avoid jock itch, a general itchy feeling in the genital area.

• Avoid applying perfume to sweaty skin. Perfume may react differently than it does on dry skin.

• To reduce sweating, exercise during the cooler hours of the day—early morning or late evening. If you prefer, exercise in an air-conditioned room.

*Scar Pains and the Weather.* Increased sunlight, especially ultraviolet light, will aggravate any pain you feel from scars.

*Jewelry and Dermatitis.* If you are sensitive to certain metals, wearing earrings may irritate or inflame your pierced ears. If so, you may buy nonmetallic (usually plastic) protective covers or "jackets" that slip over the wire posts of earrings and protect your skin from the metal.

For more information, contact:

Ms. Vicki Tartowski
2302 Newton Avenue
San Diego, CA 92113

*Eye Cosmetics.* In a study of eye cosmetics, nearly *50 percent* of the cosmetics tested were contaminated by bacteria and 10 percent by fungi! To avoid infections, discard your eye cosmetics every four months.

## Edgar Cayce Remedies

Here is an Edgar Cayce remedy called "Scar Massage," which is especially effective for acne scars and surface scar tissues.

Mix equal parts of the following and apply the oil to any scars: camphorated olive oil, witch hazel, and Russian white oil.

## For More Information

For a catalog of hypoallergenic earrings:

Roman Research Marketing
77 Accord Park Drive
Norwell, MA 02061

For information on tissue trauma and tissue healing, send a stamped, self-addressed envelope to:

Center for Tissue Trauma Research and Education
408 N.E. Alice Avenue
Jensen Beach, FL 33457

# 39

# Sleep Disorders

Sleep disorders are very common, and they have many different causes, both physical and emotional. But many people mislabel natural changes in sleeping patterns as "disorders." Therefore, before we tackle sleep disorders, let's review some of the normal ways in which sleeping patterns change.

## Your Sleeping Requirements Will Change

As you get older, you will spend less time in the deep stages of sleep. This pattern change causes many geriatric people to complain that they have insomnia, when they are simply undergoing a normal reduction in their sleep requirements.

More specifically, from age 20 to age 50, your level of deep sleep will be reduced by 60 percent. The following chart shows just how radically your sleeping requirements change as you age:

| Age Group | Average Nighttime Sleeping Hours |
|---|---|
| Newborns | 16 to 18 hours |
| Four-year-olds | 10 hours |
| Early teens | 9 hours |
| Late teens to early 20s | 7 to 8 hours |
| Age 65 and older | 4½ to 6½ hours |

Remember, too, that the elderly take more catnaps during the day, further reducing their nighttime sleep requirements. As a result, people—especially older people—often believe they are not getting enough sleep when they really *are*.

191

As one study summarized it:

> Not everyone who complains of insomnia actually suffers from it. Studies in deep-sleep laboratories reveal that many people sleep more than they think they do. Scientists estimate that at least one-third of all people who consider themselves insomniacs get as much shut-eye as people who consider themselves normal sleepers. [*Consumer Reports*, March 1987, p. 136.]

## Chart Your Sleeping Habits

Here is a simple way to check your sleeping habits. Every morning complete a chart that answers the following questions:

1. What time did I go to bed last night?
2. How many hours did I sleep?
3. Did I wake up during the night? If so, did I fall asleep a~ain easily, or did I stay awake?
4. Did I nap during the day yesterday?
5. Did I use any drugs yesterday that might have affected my sleep last night—for example, coffee, alcohol, or sleep-inducing medications?

The completed chart will tell you a lot about the quality of your sleep and whether your sleeping pattern is balanced. And don't worry if your average sleeping time seems very low, say, only five or six hours a night. Sleeping requirements may vary from four hours a night for one person to 10 hours a night for another person. As long as you are not very tired, groggy, or forgetful and you have no difficulty concentrating, do not be concerned: You may simply be one of those people who needs less sleep!

## Common Sleep Disorders

The five most common sleep disorders are:

*Hyperlixia:* An excessive amount of light sleep. Because people who suffer from this condition think that they *do* get enough sleep, hyperlixia is often difficult to recognize. Yet despite the fact that people with hyperlixia think they get enough sleep, they may still feel fatigued the next day.

*Initardia:* An inability to fall asleep promptly. Initardia is common among single people in the entertainment industry or in other so-called "glamorous" professions.

*Pleisomnia:* Sleep that is interrupted by awakening often during the night. This condition usually appears in people after age 40.

*Scurzomnia:* Short sleep. People with scurzomnia fall asleep easily but they wake up after just a few hours and are unable to fall asleep again.

*Turbula:* Sleep that is filled with unpleasant dreams, as well as the accompanying emotional discomfort that results.

## General Causes

Sleep disorders may result from a combination of several factors, rather than from one specific cause. Among the most common causes of disturbed sleep are:

• *Sleep apnea*, the repeated stoppage of breathing during the night. These occurrences, each of which can last from 25 to 125 seconds, can leave a person exhausted the next day. About 25 percent of people over age 62 experience sleep apnea. The majority of sufferers are hypertense, overweight males.

• *Depression* is a very common cause of insomnia.

• *Emotional stress and strain* contribute to sleep disorders.

• *Nutritional deficiencies*, especially low levels of certain minerals and amino acids, can contribute to sleeplessness.

• *Trauma*, such as the loss of a loved one, is a common cause of sleeplessness.

• *Weather changes*, too, affect sleeping patterns. Moderate weather may increase your need for sleep. Hot weather may decrease your need for sleep. Low-pressure weather may disturb your sleep. Extensively unstable weather conditions may also disturb your sleep.

• *Chronic aches and pains, nocturnal muscle cramps*, and the *restless leg syndrome* also contribute to sleeplessness.

## How Proper Nutrition Can Help

To promote a healthy sleeping pattern, follow this basic nutritional advice:

• Avoid alcohol and coffee, as well as all other caffeinated beverages.

• Eat your meals at the same time each day.

• Avoid eating a large meal in the evening, and always avoid eating for at least 2 hours before you go to bed.

• At your evening meal, increase your carbohydrate intake and decrease your protein intake.

• Eating high-carbohydrate foods with some fats (such as vegetable oils) may increase your level of serotonin, which helps you sleep easier.

• Be sure to eat plenty of foods rich in tryptophan—cheddar cheese, cottage cheese, whole milk, and skim milk, for example.

• Losing weight may be helpful if you suffer from sleep apnea.

## Effective Supplements

Two supplements that are especially beneficial in promoting good sleep are (1) vitamin $B_6$, which is needed to metabolize tryptophan and vitamin $B_1$, and (2) L-Tryptophan, which may ease many types of insomnia.

## Juice Therapy

For general sleep disorders, drink the juice of eight to ten celery stalks each day. Celery juice is an excellent source of magnesium, sodium, and iron.

Also try a combination of carrot juice and celery juice.

## Herbs That Help You Sleep

Among the herbs that may help you sleep are:

| | | |
|---|---|---|
| Passion flower | Valerian | Licorice |
| Hops | Oatsraw | Peppermint |
| Skullcap | Chaparral | Lady's slipper |

| Chamomile | Lobelia | Wood betony |
|-----------|---------|-------------|
| Black cohosh | Mistletoe | Capsicum |

Try one of these specific remedies:

• Use chamomile, a useful but harmless sedative. [*Journal of Clinical Pharmacology*, 1974.]

• Combine these herbs to make your own wonderful sleeping aid: valerian root, skullcap, and hops flowers.

Valerian promotes restful sleep without that groggy side effect that many sleeping aids have. Both hops and skullcap soothe the system in preparation for sleep.

• Mix this herbal formula to relieve insomnia: black cohosh, hops flowers, valerian root, cayenne, lobelia, skullcap, wood betony.

## Cranial Manipulation for Infants

Infants who bang their heads against the side of the crib or the mattress or rock the crib across the floor may be feeling pressure between the cranial bones, a pressure that results from birth trauma. Osteopathic physicians specializing in cranial manipulation are best suited to treat these children and release their cranial tension.

To locate a skilled osteopathic physician or just find out more about this therapy, contact:

Sutherland Cranial Teaching Foundation
1140 West Eighth Street
Meridian, ID 83642

## Exercise

Doing aerobic exercises regularly in the early part of the day may help you sleep better at night.

## Hydrotherapy

Try a cold sitz bath and cold, full-body sponging. Also, before bedtime try an ice massage on the back of the neck and head.

## Visualization

According to one study, a visualization technique similar to the one described on page 142 was very therapeutic in certain types of sleep disorders. [*Journal of the Royal Society of Medicine*, October, 1979.] When you use this technique, visualize yourself *sleeping*, of course.

## Homeopathy

For general insomnia, take avena sativa with lemon balm tea. In addition, here are a number of remedies for insomnia resulting from:

• *Excitement or Joy*: Coffea.

• *Mental Strain*: Nux vomica.

• *Anxiety or Worry*: Arsenicum.

• *Nervousness*: Salix nig. and passiflora.

## Tissue Salts

For insomnia accompanied by nervousness, try potassium phosphate.

## General Sleeping Tips

Following these suggestions may help you improve the quality and the quantity of your sleeping time:

1. Take a warm bath or warm shower about half an hour before you go to bed.

2. Go to bed at the same time each evening. If you feel wide awake and cannot fall asleep immediately, adapt the visualization technique described on page 142. In Step #4, visualize yourself *sleeping*. If you prefer, listen to calm, soothing music. Do not try to "make up for" lost sleep on weekends or holidays.

3. Wake up at a specific preset time each morning, even if you did not sleep well the night before. In other words, don't sleep later in an effort to make up for lost sleep. After a night or more of sleeplessness, you *will* probably sleep longer and better.

4. Except for making love and meditating, in bed, do nothing other than sleep.

5. If you are lying in bed awake for 30 minutes, get up and walk around for a few minutes or do something else—something *boring*. Do *not* eat, watch TV, or read a good book. After a few minutes, go back to bed.

6. Many different relaxation techniques are effective in relieving insomnia, including autogenic training, deep breathing, visualization, self-hypnosis, and progressive relaxation.

7. To a glass of buttermilk, add two tablespoons of honey and the juice of one lemon. Drink this mixture before you retire.

8. Use a pillow filled with loose, natural material. Such pillows "breathe" to stay cool and dry; at the same time, they are soft and yet offer firm support. If you are allergic to natural fibers, try a pillow filled with buckwheat hulls. Used in Japan for centuries, these pillows are generally hypoallergenic. In the United States, these pillows are available under the brand name "Alpha Pillow."

9. Follow the nutrition tips listed on page 193.

10. Exercise!

## Specific Remedies

Try these remedies for specific sleeping problems:

*For Snoring:* Often considered annoying but harmless, in some people snoring may indicate a collapse of the soft tissue at the top of the windpipe and possibly a higher risk of heart attack than people who do not snore. As the tongue, the tonsils, and other soft tissue totally block the windpipe, they cut off oxygen, forcing the body to work much harder to get air. Blood pressure and heart abnormalities may result, leading to heart attacks.

One remedy is to wear the TRD device described here in "Sleep Apnea."

*For Sleep Apnea:* Instead of surgery, long the only treatment for sleep apnea, the modern therapy is simply wearing a special appliance called a "tongue-retaining device" or "TRD." This device holds your tongue in a forward position while you sleep, preventing your tongue from obstructing your air passages. [*Journal of the American Medical Association*, August 13, 1982.]

Very obviously, wearing a TRD is much preferred over surgery.

## For More Information

A very helpful organization for information about sleep disorders is the Association of Sleep Disorder Centers (ASDC):

ASDC
P.O. Box 2604
Del Mar, CA 92014

# 40

# Stress

Of all your body's systems, the nervous system is the most fragile. Its delicate balance is easily affected by emotional, physical, or chemical factors, or by a combination of these factors. As a result of an imbalance, you may suffer from stress, insomnia, nervous tension, and a host of other disorders.

Here we are concerned with *stress*, a term first used by the renowned researcher on the subject, Dr. Hans Selye of the University of Montreal's Institute of Experimental Medicine, to describe specific body reactions to certain stimuli.

## When Stress Is Beneficial

Although we may tend to automatically consider stress and tension as harmful, they are essential parts of our everyday lives and are actually necessary for a balanced, productive existence. Consider, for example, the fact that both sex and laughter create a certain amount of stress and then provide a release of stress.

Stress may even help fight cancer. Research studies show that the body reacts to stress by increasing "its production of natural opiates called beta-endorphines, which appear to stimulate antitumor lymphocytes. These cells aid the body in fighting cancer by their role in activating the body's immune system." [Richard D. Lyons, "Stress Addiction: 'Life in the Fast Lane' May Have Its Benefits," *New York Times*, July 26, 1983, Section C, p. 9.]

So you see that stress *can* be beneficial, but only in moderate quantities.

## When Stress Is Harmful

Stress in immoderate quantities, on the other hand, overloads the body's resources and can be very harmful. If the body cannot handle the stress overload, it may react with a "pathological" tension. When this tension increases, your breathing may become very shallow. Shallow breathing has a pronounced effect on the blood circulation throughout the body and reduces the amount of oxygen that reaches the brain. In addition to shallow breathing, your muscles will tighten up, especially around your pelvis, neck, and shoulders.

This abnormal tension and reduced circulation are associated with a number of disorders, including:

| | |
|---|---|
| Aches and pains | Diarrhea |
| Certain types of arthritis | Sexual problems |
| Alcoholism | Mood swings |
| Asthma | Lethargy |
| Backache | Reduced immunological function |
| Canker sores | Insomnia |
| Headaches | Dermatitis and other skin disorders |
| Hypertension | Colitis, ulcers, and other |
| Cardiovascular disease | gastrointestinal disorders |
| Diabetes | |

Trying to eliminate all stress and tension is both impractical and impossible, but there certainly are ways to minimize their effects, as we will see in this section.

## Are *You* a High-Stress Person?

You are probably a high-stress person if you:

- Eat, move about, and usually walk rapidly.
- Speak very quickly and rush through the ends of your sentences.
- Are impatient.
- Cannot relax without feeling guilty about not working or not taking care of something important.
- Think about work while on vacation.
- Usually try to do two things at once.
- Believe *time management* means "doing more things in less time."
- Are in love with your own opinion and do not listen to the opinions of others.
- Define success in terms of how quickly you accomplish things.
- Place greater emphasis on owning or controlling things, rather than *enjoying* them.

## The Role of Nutrition

Following the general nutritional recommendations in this book—especially the suggestions offered in the sections on "Cardiovascular Disease" and "Hypertension"—will help you cope with tension and stress.

Be especially sure to avoid coffee, tea, alcohol, tobacco, refined and processed foods, sugar, flour, white rice, and so on.

## Supplements That Help

Magnesium depletion has been associated with high-stress personalities, people who exhibit what is called "Type A" behavior. Magnesium deficiency is also considered a factor in hypertension and certain cardiovascular diseases.

Magnesium is especially beneficial for high-stress people because magnesium helps the muscles to relax. Be sure to review the suggestions for supplements in the section on "Hypertension," which begins on page 101.

## Amino Acid Therapy

GABA (gamma-aminobutryic acid) may reduce acute agitation due to stress and increase your level of calmness and tranquility by inhibiting neurotransmitters.

## Juice Therapy

According to N. W. Walker, the pioneer of juice therapy:

> The juice of Romaine Lettuce, with the addition of a small amount of kelp (seaweed), has been found to contain properties conducive to helping the activity of the Adrenal Cortex in its function of secreting its hormone, Adrenaline, to keep the body in balance. [N. W. Walker, *Raw Vegetable Juices*, New York, Pyramid Books, 1976, p. 69.]

In addition, try mixing romaine lettuce half-and-half with carrot juice. Drink 16 ounces of this mixture twice a day.

## Herbs That Are Especially Effective

Among the herbs that are beneficial in fighting stress are:

| | |
|---|---|
| Siberian ginseng | Mistletoe |
| Black cohosh | Passion flower |
| Chamomile | Skullcap |
| Hops | Wood betony |
| Capsicum | Valerian root |
| Lady's slipper | Vervain |
| Lobelia | Catnip |

Siberian ginseng, in particular, is a first-rate stress fighter.

## Aroma Therapy

Impregnate absorbant cotton with the following essences and inhale deeply:

- Chamomile and melissa—antispasmodics and nerve sedatives.
- Lavender, geranium, and patchouli—for tension and anxiety.

Other plant essences that have long been used to reduce stress, nervous disability, mental fatigue, anxiety, and tension include:

| | | |
|---|---|---|
| Basil | Borneo camphor | Clove |
| Bergamot | Cinnamon | Cypress |

| Eucalyptus | Lemon | Rosemary |
| Garlic | Nutmeg | Marjoram |
| Geranium | Onion | Neroli |
| Ginger | Peppermint | Rose |
| Hyssop | Pine | Thyme |
| Lavender | | |

## Acupressure and Massage

Use deep rhythmic pressure on the stress release points, as described in the Appendix.

## Exercise to Release Stress

Try these techniques to release stress through exercising:

1. Clench your fists as tightly as possible for about 5 seconds, then release them. Now shake your hands loosely.

2. To relieve headaches and tension around the forehead, raise and lower your eyebrows as quickly as possible while you keep your head still and focus your eyes straight ahead.

3. To relieve eye stress and tension, open your eyes as wide as you can and then squeeze them together as tight as you can. Repeat this process three or four times throughout the day.

4. Perform some range-of-motion exercises.

5. Practice yoga or stretching exercises.

6. Walk briskly or swim laps for one-half hour three times a week.

7. Use an exercise videotape as you perform aerobic exercises indoors. If you prefer, use a trampoline or other form of rebounding apparatus.

8. Not exactly an "exercise," but perhaps you might find this helpful to release your emotional frustrations: Hit your bed or your pillow. Raise both your arms over your head and clench your fists tightly. Then hit the bed or the pillow with your forearms and fists at the same time.

## Hydrotherapy

Try the following hydrotherapy techniques to relieve stress:

- Alternate hot and cold showers.
- Take a hot Epsom salt bath.
- Try seawater baths (thalasotherapy).
- Take a hot chamomile flower footbath.

## Homeopathy

*For Nervous Temperament:* Ignatia.
*To Relieve Stress:* Phosphoric acid.
*For General Nervousness:* Agnus castus and passiflora.
Also try the Bach Flower Remedies. See page 230.

## Visualization

Use the two visualization techniques described on (1) page 142 and (2) page 151 to relieve stress. In addition, try this visualization technique for a basic approach to relaxation:

Step 1. Find a quiet place where you will not be disturbed. Sit in a straight-back chair with both your feet flat on the floor and place your hands, palms up, on your knees.

Step 2. Close your eyes. Inhale and exhale long and slowly.

Step 3. As you exhale, visualize that you are actually exhaling the stress and the tension from your body.

Step 4. Complete your visualization by (a) taking a long, deep breath, (b) slowly exhaling, and (c) gradually opening your eyes. Sit quietly for a few minutes as you become aware once again of your surroundings.

Step 5. Slowly begin to wiggle your fingers and toes. Rise only when you feel acclimated to your surroundings.

## Also of Interest

Note the following:

• The most popular ways to overcome stress are relaxation training, visualization techniques, exercising, biofeedback training, and finding a quiet, secluded place whenever you are surrounded with noise, smoke, or too many people.

• When you are confronted with the stress of loneliness, call someone for a chat—a friend, a colleague, a coworker, anyone with whom you can discuss an idea you have or a problem you've been working on.

• Develop close, personal, supportive relationships. If you find the idea of giving up your independence frightening, perhaps you should consider professional counseling.

• Take 3-minute breaks throughout your workday. If you can find a place to lie down, raise your feet above your head and relax.

• Listen to quiet, soothing music whenever possible. Use a portable cassette player.

• Take a short walk from time to time.

• Take a 15-minute nap.

• Do deep-breathing and relaxation exercises.

• Register for a time-management class.

• Use stress-reduction tools on the job—for example, reflexology sandals, biofeedback indicators (strips, dots, rings), and so on.

# 41

# Urinary Tract Disorders

Disorders involving the kidneys and the urinary tract include:

- Cystitis
- Infections
- Hypertension (high blood pressure)
- Inflammation of the kidneys (nephritis)
- Kidney stones
- Kidney failure
- Bleeding (caused by kidney malfunction)

The two leading causes of kidney failure are high blood pressure and diabetes, in that order.

## Cystitis

Cystitis is an infection marked by an inflammation of the urinary bladder. Its symptoms include a constant feeling of the need to urinate, extreme pain while urinating, and blood in the urine.

There are many causes of cystitis, including:

- Bacterial infection (the same bacterium that causes vaginitis), either (a) passed on by a male sexual partner or (b) transmitted in the course of wiping the anus after a bowel movement.

- A kidney infection that has traveled down to the bladder.
- Frequent intercourse, or intercourse after a long abstinence.
- Certain vaginal deodorants.
- Food allergies.
- Uterine prolapse.
- Infrequent urination or withholding urinating for too long a time.

Cystitis affects women more often than it affects men, perhaps because bacteria travel more easily through the shorter female urethra.

## Kidney Stones: What Are They?

The kidneys serve as the body's waste-disposal system. A *kidney stone* is an obstruction in this system. The stone itself may be any size, a small as a pinhead or as large as a grapefruit. It may be any shape. It may be rough or smooth.

About 10 percent of all kidney stones result from general metabolism problems or from specific problems with the kidney itself. The other 90 percent probably result from an imbalance in the urine, although not much is known about this imbalance. In any case, before effective therapy can begin, the chemical makeup or composition of the stone must be determined.

## Kidney Stones: What Causes Them?

The known causes of kidney stones include:

- Structural problems in the kidneys that result in poor urine drainage.
- Cysts in the middle of the kidney that inhibit urine flow.
- Birth defects that result in chemical imbalances in the urine and contribute to stone formation.
- Various metabolic disorders, including excessive intestinal absorption of oxalates, gouty arthritis, and hyperparathyroidism, a condition that leads to too much calcium in the blood and urine.
- Excessive consumption of milk, milk products, and vitamin D.

## Kidney Stones: What Are They Made Of?

As we said earlier, knowing the composition of stones is important for treatment. Common kidney stones are made up of:

1. Calcium oxalate.
2. Calcium oxalate surrounding a core of uric acid.
3. Calcium phosphate.
4. A combination of calcium oxalate and calcium phosphate.

Often, kidney stones pose enough problems to require surgical removal, but many stones require no treatment at all. They may pass out of the kidney during urination (with considerable pain), or they may remain in the kidney, causing no harm and no symptoms.

## Nephritis

Nephritis, an inflammation of one or both kidneys, may be characterized by a number
of symptoms:

| | |
|---|---|
| Anemia | Loss of appetite |
| A frequent urge to urinate | Vomiting |
| Nausea | Swelling |
| Chills | Abdominal pain |
| Fatigue | Lower-back pain |
| Blood in the urine | |

*Pyelonephritis.* Pyelonephritis, the most common type of nephritis, is caused by
an infection in the urinary opening and usually affects women during pregnancy or
childbirth. The bacteria may be passed to the urinary opening after a bowel movement
if the rectum is wiped in a forward, rather than a backward, motion.

*Glomerulonephritis.* This type of nephritis is usually a reaction to an infection
elsewhere in the body.

## Pyelitis

Pyelitis is an inflammation of the kidney passages.

### The Role of Nutrition in Renal Insufficiency

In cases of renal insufficiency, the patient may be able to avoid a dialysis machine if he
or she follows a special diet. The results of a recent research study indicate that "a
low-protein, low-phosphorus diet supplemented with amino acids and keto acids can
markedly influence the course of progressive chronic renal failure, as indicated by
changes in the serum creatinine level." [*Harvard Medical Area Focus*, December 6,
1984, p. 1. *New England Journal of Medicine*, September 6, 1984, pp. 623-628.]

For more information about this new nutritional approach to renal insufficiency,
contact:

Harvard Medical Area News Office
25 Shattuck Street
Boston, MA 02115
(617) 732-1590

### How Nutrition Can Help in General Disorders

For general disorders of the urinary tract, including kidney and bladder disorders, follow these recommendations:

• Follow a vegetarian diet that is low in protein and high in complex carbohydrates. Be sure to include plenty of steamed vegetables, raw fruits, salads, brown rice,
and raw, certified goat's milk. You may also include yogurt, kefir, and other cultured-
milk products.

• Eat frequent small meals.

• Avoid salt.

• Be sure to eat the foods that are considered most effective in healing urinary tract infections: parsley, watercress, celery, horseradish, asparagus, cucumber, potatoes, watermelon.

## How Nutrition Can Help in Specific Conditions

Here are a number of recommendations for specific disorders.

*Kidney Stones.* Your nutritional habits can help treat kidney stones:

1. Contrary to old myths, cutting down on calcium intake over a long period of time does *not* reduce the potential for stone formation. Worse, the cutback in calcium may contribute to bone loss and osteoporosis.

2. Using significant amounts of sugar and sugar products can increase your chances of calcium stone formation. If you have a history of forming stones, avoid foods high in oxalates including spinach, unhulled sesame seeds, chocolate, beets, pepper, rhubarb, tea, nuts, and figs.

3. If you have calcium phosphate stones, avoid very concentrated alkaline foods, such as fruit juices and cola-based soft drinks. If the stone formation is associated with gout, be sure to drink a lot of fluids—three to four quarts daily—to reduce uric acid concentrations in your system.

4. Increase your intake of high-fiber foods to reduce your chances of stone formation. People who produce large amounts of uric acid are susceptible to uric acid stones. Generally, these people consume large amounts of animal protein—meat, fish, and poultry—and do not use many high-fiber foods.

5. Lower your intake of high-fat foods. People with high-fat intakes have higher stone formation.

6. Lower your intake of milk and milk products.

*Nephritis.* Reduce your protein intake.

## Supplements That Help

Supplements can help you clear up urinary tract disorders:

*Cystitis.* Take vitamin C in ascorbic acid form.

*Kidney Disease.* Take ¼ ounce of activated charcoal three times a day for four weeks to lower blood-fat levels. This therapy worked very effectively in a recent Finnish study. [*The Lancet*, August 16, 1986.]

People with kidney disease are very sensitive to increased blood fat and the risk of atherosclerosis, one of the major causes of death among long-term dialysis patients. People with failing kidneys cannot metabolize lipids, *fats*, in a normal way. Activated charcoal may reduce this risk. [*Men's Health*, February 1987, p. 7.]

*Kidney Failure.* Supplement with carnitine.

*Kidney Stones.* Several supplements are effective in avoiding kidney stones, and others are best avoided, as explained here:

• *Magnesium and Vitamin $B_6$.* Magnesium helps prevent stone formation by dissolving oxalic acid, a major cause of stone formation, in the urine. Also, vitamin $B_6$ significantly lowers the oxalate content in the urine. [*International Journal of Clinical Pharmacology, Therapy, and Toxicology*, 1982.]

Furthermore, magnesium and vitamin $B_6$ *in combination* reduce the potential for calcium oxalate stone formation even more.

Also, reduce your calcium intake to the recommended daily allowance and avoid taking calcium supplementation. Many nutritionists also recommend taking 500 milligrams of magnesium oxide daily.

• *Vitamin C.* If your vitamin C intake is too high, you may develop an unusually high oxalate level and contribute to stone formation. your physician can test the oxalate levels in your urine as follows:

For about three weeks, take a high level of vitamin C (say, 8 to 10 grams). Do not take any other vitamins during this time.

Collect urine samples for 24 hours. Your doctor will send this sample to a lab for a "24-hour urinary oxalate excretion test."

The normal oxalate level in urine is 40 milligrams or less within a 24-hour period. If your oxalate level is higher, (1) reduce your intake of vitamin C or (2) supplement with 100 milligrams of vitamin $B_6$, which will prevent vitamin C from inducing oxalate formation.

*Nephritis.* Note these recommendations for people suffering from nephritis:

1. Reduce your intake of potassium and sodium to the Recommended Daily Allowance.

2. If you are anemic, take an iron supplement.

3. Supplement with vitamin C. Even in severe cases of nephritis, patients had good results when they supplemented with 5,000 milligrams of vitamin C plus 500 milligrams of bioflavonoid complex.

*Urinary Tract Infection.* To heal urinary tract infections, follow these suggestions:

1. Take 3,000 milligrams of vitamin C each day. [*New York State Journal of Medicine*, December 15, 1971.]

2. Drink this combination with each meal: To a glass of warm distilled water, add two teaspoons of apple cider vinegar and one teaspoon of honey. This mixture will help acidify the urine.

3. Reduce your intake of fruits and vegetables to a minimum. These foods are very alkaline and may interfere with the healing process in the acute state of the infection. Instead, follow a macrobiotic-type diet, eating plenty of seeds, nuts, and grains. But keep your intake of miso, soy sauce, and sea salt to a minimum.

Children with urinary tract infections should avoid cow's milk, which can cause constipation and further aggravate the condition.

## Juice Therapy

The first choice in juice therapy for urinary tract infections is unsweetened cranberry juice. In the early acute stages of kidney or bladder infection, avoid most fruit and vegetable juices, because they are too alkaline and may actually aggravate the condition.

In addition, note these specific uses of juices (all the Juice Therapy Formulas mentioned are listed in the Appendix):

*For General Kidney Problems:* For albuminuria, nephritis, and calculi of the kidney and bladder, try these effective remedies:

• A combination of these juices: carrot, asparagus, and parsley.

- Juice Therapy Formula #2.
- Any *one* of these healing juices: watermelon, cucumber, or celery.
- Add watercress and garlic to carrot juice and drink this combination.

*For Cystitis and Other Bladder Disorders:* Juice Therapy Formulas #6 and #17. Also, drink unsweetened cranberry juice.

*For Kidney Stones:* Juice Therapy Formula #6.

*As a Diuretic:* Juice Therapy Formulas #4 and #5. When not combined with other juices, cucumber juice is one of the strongest and most effective natural diuretics.

*For Urinary Tract Infections:* Drink cranberry juice for the first few days. Then, as symptoms improve, start drinking carrot juice.

## Herbal Remedies

Several herbal remedies are especially effective for urinary tract conditions:

*For General Kidney Disorders:* Try a combination of these herbs: goldenrod, bedstraw, and yellow dead nettle. Other healing herbs for urinary tract infections are corn silk, dandelion, juniper berries, parsley, garlic, buchu, shepherd's purse, uva ursi, catnip, asparagus, and goldenseal.

*For Cystitis:* Mix these herbs: plantain, slippery elm, ginger, and uva ursi. Another remedy is to take goldenseal root, chaparral, and echinacea in tablets or in rice paper.

*For Kidney Stones:* Mix the following herbs:

4 parts Gravel root
4 parts Parsley root
4 parts Marsh Mallow root
1 part Lobelia
1 part Ginger root

Boil this mixture for 20 to 30 minutes. Then strain the herbs. Drink ½ cup three times a day.

## Aroma Therapy

Aroma therapy can be very effective in treating urinary tract disorders:

*For General Urinary Tract Disorders:* The most effective essences are juniper, sage, and thyme—especially against *Staphyloccocus aureus* infections. These three essences are also powerful diuretics.

*For Dissolving Urinary Stones:* Chamomile and geranium oils are effective for dissolving urinary stones. Apply these oils by hip bath, by local compresses, and by massaging the lumbar and sacral area. You may also take chamomile and geranium orally.

Fennel, garlic, geranium, hyssop, juniper, and lemon are also effective essences for dissolving urinary stones.

*For Cystitis:* Use these essences: cajeput, eucalyptus, fennel, juniper, lavender, niaouli, pine, sandalwood, thuja, thyme.

*As a Diuretic:* Essences of cypress, juniper, onion, rosemary, sage, and thyme.

*For Gallstones:* To prevent the formation of gallstones, as well as to treat them, try these essences: lemon, nutmeg, onion, pine, and rosemary.

*For Urinary Tract Infections:* Sandalwood is a specific disinfectant for urinary tract infections. Other powerful essences include juniper, lavender, niaouli, onion, and thyme.

## Acupressure and Massage

For urinary tract disorders, lymphatic kneading is very effective, as well as circular rhythmic pressure (see the Appendix). Also, see the suggestion for dissolving urinary stones under "Aroma Therapy."

## Hydrotherapy

Several hydrotherapy procedures can be effective in treating urinary tract disorders.

*General Kidney Problems:* For general problems associated with kidneys, try these hydrotherapy techniques (all are discussed in the Appendix):

- Upper-body sponging
- High-pressure cold-water shower on the knees
- Cold-sheet wrapping

For an effective diuretic, apply an onion poultice to the kidneys and lower abdomen.

*Cystitis:* Try steam baths and full-body cold-water sponging. See the Appendix.

*Stones:* Apply warm castor oil packs over the kidneys.

## Homeopathy for Pyelitis

Pyelitis is an inflammation of the kidney passages. If your symptoms include swelling, chills, fever, and scanty urination, use apis. If your symptoms include deep pains at the waist, then use berberis.

## Tissue Salts

For cystitis, use potassium chloride, phosphate of iron, and calcium sulfate.

## General Suggestions for Preventing Cystitis

To avoid the chances of getting cystitis, see pages 202 and 203.

## Also of Interest

In West Germany, a machine called a *Lithotripter* uses shock waves to pulverize kidney stones, avoiding the need for surgery. Once pulverized, the stones pass through the body easily.

## Susan B. Gets Permanent Relief From Bladder Infection

For years, Susan B. was plagued by recurrent bladder infections. She suffered from lower-back pain in the evenings, and she felt a burning sensation during urination. In the past, she felt temporary relief with antibiotics, but the pain returned soon after she stopped the medication.

Finally, two years ago, Susan found *lasting* relief when she began a program that included:

- Drinking (1) apple cider vinegar in water daily, (2) cranberry juice three times a day, and (3) distilled water with Megadophilus (a brand of acidophilus).

- Douching with apple cider vinegar mixed with Megadophilus.
- Supplementing with vitamins $B_6$ and C.
- Taking hot sitz baths every evening.
- Applying warm castor oil packs over the kidney area.

Now, two years after she began following this program, Susan has had no recurrence of bladder infection.

# Appendix

# APPENDIX A

# Juice Therapy

## Juice Therapy Techniques

Juices are essential catalysts that allow the body to heal. Perhaps the key to juice therapy is the amount of *enzymes* available in fresh juices. Enzymes perform many biological processes and greatly assist your digestive function, assimiliation, and elimination.

Throughout this book, various juice therapy formulas are recommended as remedies for specific conditions or disorders. The recipe for each of the formulas referred to in this book is listed on pages 213 and 214. As you apply these formulas, be sure to follow these general suggestions:

1. Drink only freshly extracted juices. Canned and bottled juices are of limited value—or *no* value—in a juice therapy program.

2. Drink juices immediately after you extract them. Do not refrigerate or store juice for later use.

3. Be sure to use *fresh* fruits and vegetables. Green vegetables should not be pale, they should have full color. Avoid iceberg lettuce, blanched celery, and so on.

4. Drink about 16 ounces of juice a day if you are generally healthy. If you are not in general good health, you may need to drink 16-ounce portions of juice at least two to four times a day. Specific quantities will vary according to the treatment.

*Formula #1:* 8 oz. carrot, 8 oz. apple, 5 oz. beet, 5 oz. cucumber

*Formula #2:* 8 oz. carrot, 8 oz. celery, 8 oz. parsley

*Formula #3:* 10 oz. carrot, 3 oz. celery, 3 oz. cabbage

*Formula #4:* 6 oz. cabbage, 6 oz. cucumber, 4 oz. grapefruit
NOTE: Formula #4 is not recommended for people suffering from colitis.

*Formula #5:* 14 oz. carrot, ½ lemon, squeezed, ½ tspn. horseradish root, grated. Mix the horseradish root into the carrot juice, then add the lemon juice.

*Formula #6:* 6 oz. carrot, 5 oz. cucumber, 5 oz. beet

*Formula #7:* 4 oz. apple, 4 oz. carrot, 4 oz. celery, 2 oz. beet, 2 oz. spinach

*Formula #8:* carrot, celery, beet and beet tops, alfalfa sprouts

*Formula #9:* pear, kale, carrot, asparagus, cucumber

*Formula #10:* 10 oz. cucumber, 4 oz. carrot, 2 oz. raw potato

*Formula #11:* 7 oz. carrot, 5 oz. green pepper

*Formula #12:* 7 oz. carrot, 6 oz. cucumber, 2 oz. parsley

*Formula #13:* 5 oz. Brussels sprout, 5 oz. string bean, 2 oz. carrot, 2 oz. escarole

*Formula #14:* 7 oz. escarole, 6 oz. carrot, 3 oz. celery

*Formula #15:* 6 oz. cucumber, 4 oz. carrot, 3 oz. parsley, 2 oz. beet

*Formula #16:* 10 oz. carrot, 3 oz. dandelion, 3 oz. turnip leaves

*Formula #17:* 6 oz. carrot, 4 oz. watercress, 3 oz. spinach, 3 oz. turnip leaves

*Formula #18:* 4 large- or medium-size grapefruits, 3 medium-size lemons, 3 quarts distilled water

Note: Formula #18, a modified version of one of N. W. Walker's formulas, helps restore the body's alkalinity and cleanses the lymphatic system. Take about six ounces every 30 minutes until you finish the entire mixture. At the end of the day, drink a glass of celery and carrot juices, combined. Continue this for two or three days. At the end of the three-day period, begin a raw food diet.

*Formula #19:* 7 oz. carrot, 4 oz. celery, 3 oz. spinach, 2 oz. parsley

*Formula #20:* 10 oz. carrot, 6 oz. spinach

*Formula #21:* 6 oz. carrots, 6 oz. cucumbers, 4 oz. celery, 4 oz. beets

*Formula #22:* 6 oz. carrots, 6 oz. spinach, 4 oz. celery

*Formula #23:* 8 oz. carrots, 2 oz. cucumbers, 6 oz. celery

*Formula #24:* 16 oz. carrots, 16 oz. celery

*Formula #25:* 8 oz. green leafy vegetable juice, 8 oz. beet juice, 1 oz. dandelion juice

## Specific Benefits of Juices

The key nutrients in juices, as well as many of their most important uses, are listed here:

*Apple:* Pectin, potassium, phosphorus, and cellulose.

*Asparagus:* An effective diuretic, asparagus juice is very healing to the kidneys. It is especially valuable for breaking up oxalic acid accumulation.

*Beet:* Potassium. Beet juice is used to build blood.

*Beet Greens:* Vitamin A, potassium, calcium, and iron.

*Blueberry:* Used as an astringent, antiseptic, and blood purifier.

*Brussels Sprout:* Regenerates pancreatic function and digestion.

*Cabbage:* Sulfur, chlorine, and iodine. A great cleanser for the mucous membranes of the intestines and the stomach.

*Carrot:* Beta-carotene, potassium, sodium, calcium, magnesium, and iron. Carrot juice is the greatest source of beta-carotene of all juices. It is a powerful aid to the maintenance of bones and teeth and is especially valuable for disorders of the liver and intestines.

*Celery:* Potassium, sodium, calcium, phosphorus, and magnesium.

*Cucumber:* Chlorine, sulfur, silicon. Probably the most powerful diuretic of all juices.

*Dandelion:* Potassium, calcium, sodium, magnesium, and iron. Dandelion juice is used to counteract hyperacidity in the system.

*Fennel:* A powerful blood builder.

*Garlic:* Extremely rich in mustard oils, garlic is a powerful cleanser for mucus in the sinus cavities and the bronchial tubes. For best results, mix garlic with other, milder juices.

*Grapefruit:* Vitamin C and potassium.

*Kale:* Kale is used in the same way as cabbage juice.

*Leek:* Leek is used the same way as garlic or onion juice, but leek is much milder.

*Lemon:* Vitamin C and bioflavonoids. Lemon juice is a powerful cleanser of the mucus.

*Onion:* Used the same way as garlic, but onion juice is much milder.

*Parsnip:* (cultivated, not wild parsnip) Chlorine, potassium, phosphorus, silicon, and sulfur.

*Papaya:* Although ripe papaya is delicious, *un*ripe papaya is high in papain, a protein-digesting enzyme. According to N. W. Walker, a pioneer of juice therapy, the juice of unripe papaya also contains fibrin, an element that is valuable for coagulating or clotting the blood.

*Parsley:* Vitamin C, vitamin A, calcium, and magnesium.

*Potato:* Chlorine, phosphorus, potassium, and sulfur.

*Radish:* Potassium, sodium, iron, and magnesium.

*Sorrel:* Iron, magnesium, phosphorus, sulfur, and silicon.

*Tomato:* Sodium, calcium, potassium, and magnesium.

*Turnip:* Turnip leaves may have the highest level of calcium of all juicing vegetables.

*Watercress:* Sulfur, phosphorus, and chlorine.

# APPENDIX B

# Hydrotherapy Techniques

## Uses and Benefits of Hydrotherapy

Hydrotherapy offers many specific benefits for treating certain conditions. For example, hydrotherapy:

- Increases blood circulation.
- Selectively raises or lowers body temperature.
- Stimulates the activity of the internal organs (this increased activity, in turn, increases metabolic processes and helps drain waste products).
- Promotes or restores normal skin activity.
- Increases muscle function, relaxes tight muscles, develops muscle tone, and relieves muscle pain due to cramps and spasm.
- Reduces inflammation.
- Reduces swelling.
- Stops bleeding.
- Relieves constipation.

The hydrotherapy techniques recommended in this book are explained in detail.

## Cold Packs and Compresses

Proceed as follows:

1. Take a towel or facecloth made of cotton (or some other natural fiber) and dip it into very cold water—water to which you have added a few ice cubes. Fold the moist towel *twice* to create four layers.

2. Place the moistened towel on the area to be treated.

3. Cover the compress with a dry folded towel. Make sure that the dry towel completely covers the wet area, and be sure to avoid drafts. If you wish, cover the bed with a rubber sheet before you begin to make sure that no water gets into the mattress.

4. After about 10 minutes, redip the cloth in the cold water and repeat the process for 1 hour.

5. After 1 hour, remove the wet compress, dry yourself and cover yourself fully. Do not expose the wet area too long.

NOTES:

1. Moist compresses are very useful for increasing circulation and removing impurities through the skin.

2. When placing a cold compress on the eyes, use a small handkerchief or a washcloth.

3. Do *not* reuse a cloth unless you have boiled it after each use.

## Cold-Sheet Wrapping

You may need someone to assist you with this technique to ensure that you are not exposed to a draft. Proceed as follows:

1. Cover your bed with a plastic or a rubber sheet.

2. Take a wool blanket, fold it in two, and place the blanket on the plastic sheet.

3. Take a bedsheet about 9 feet long and fold it *twice* to make four layers. The folded sheet should reach from under your armpits to your knees.

4. Soak the folded bedsheet in cold water, then wring it out so that it is still moist, but not dripping wet.

5. Spread the wet bedsheet on top of the blanket. Allow the blanket to extend past the sheet about 1 inch on the top and the bottom.

6. Undress yourself and lie down on the wet sheet. Position yourself so that the upper edge of the sheet reaches your armpits.

7. Fold the wet sheet closely onto your body so that both sides of the sheet overlap and allow no draft to enter.

8. Fold the blanket around you in the same way, but not too tightly.

9. Pull a pajama top over your arms and tuck it in. In this way, you can keep your arms outside the cold sheet.

10. Pull the regular bedcovers up to your armpits, or if you prefer, to your chin. Be sure to tuck in the bedcovers all around, even under your shoulder blades.

11. Lie still in this cold-sheet wrapping for 45 minutes. Then redip the sheet in cold water and rewrap yourself once again, following the same procedure outlined in steps 4 through 10 above.

12. After the second wrapping, remove the sheets and blankets, but do not dry yourself. Put on pajamas, cover yourself well, and stay in bed for about 40 minutes.

13. Change into dry pajamas, get in bed again, and cover yourself well.

## High-Pressure Cold-Water Shower

High-pressure cold-water showers are especially valuable for treating infections of the legs, arms, and fingers. Using a shower-massage unit or a high-pressure shower with the head removed, proceed as follows:

1. Stand in the shower stall or bathtub. Set the water to the coldest setting and spray the area to be treated. If you are using a shower-massage unit or a hose, hold the

end of the unit about 3 inches away. Angle the spray so that the water pours onto you like a sheet, rather than in single streams or trickles.

2. Without drying yourself, wrap yourself in a dry bath towel and cover yourself with a warm blanket.

Alternating hot and cold showers may also be very beneficial. Proceed as follows:

1. Begin with warm or hot water.
2. Stay under the warm- or hot-water spray for two to three minutes.
3. Slowly change the temperature setting from hot to cool or cold water.
4. Remain under the cold water for 30 seconds.
5. Alternate between hot and cold as described in Steps 1 to 4 above.
6. *Always* finish with cold water.
7. Dry yourself vigorously and cover yourself quickly to avoid any drafts.

NOTE: High-pressure cold-water and hot-water showers are not recommended in cases of:

- Asthma
- Heart trouble
- High blood pressure
- Thrombosis of the coronary arteries

## Upper-Body Sponging

For upper-body sponging, proceed as follows:

1. In a warm, draft-free room, fill a basin with very cold water.
2. Wrap and tuck a thick bath towel around your waist. Keep another towel handy; you will need it later.
3. Remove your clothing above the waist.
4. Dip a facecloth in the cold water and begin washing the upper part of your body in quick, even strokes, dipping the facecloth frequently.
5. Follow this specific sequence:

Back of the shoulders toward the waist (as far as you can reach, or have someone help you).

Front of the shoulders toward the waist.

Beneath the right arm, moving from the fingertips toward the shoulder. Then return downward on the outside of the arm.

Repeat the previous step on the left arm.

6. Without drying yourself, wrap the second bath towel around your shoulders and remove the towel from your waist.
7. Now get in bed and pull the covers up to your chin to avoid any draft.
8. After about 30 minutes, put your clothes on, but do not go outdoors for at least another 30 minutes.

## Footbaths

For poor circulation of the feet, use *lukewarm* water. Although hot water increases the metabolism of the legs under normal conditions, if your circulation is poor, your system may not be strong enough to meet the increased need for blood. Thus hot water can do more harm than good. Obviously, very cold water can further decrease circulation and can cause further damage, especially in diabetics.

## Sitz Baths

*With Tepid Water.* Use neutral or tepid water for sitz baths for the following conditions: prostate trouble (in elderly men), fatigue and exhaustion, asthma, and heart trouble.

Proceed as follows:

1. Stay under a blanket in a warm bed for about 30 minutes.

2. Fill the bathtub with either hot or cold water, depending on the purpose of the treatment.

3. Remove the bottom part of your pajamas. Leave the top part on, but roll the top part up as far as possible.

4. Sit in the bathtub. Dangle your legs over the side of the tub. Do not submerge your legs or your upper body in the water.

5. Count from *1* to *50*. (Say "*one*, two, three, four," "*two*, two, three, four," "*three*, two three, four," and so on.)

6. Stand up in the tub and shake off the water. Do not dry yourself.

7. Wrap a very large bath towel around your hips and tuck in the ends firmly. Then roll down your pajama top.

8. Lie in bed as quickly as possible. Be sure to cover yourself well to avoid any drafts.

9. Stay in bed for one hour.

*With Alternating Hot and Cold Water.* You may benefit by alternating between hot and cold sitz baths for certain conditions such as delayed or painful menstruation, low sexual desire, hemorrhoids, and inflammation around the genitals.

Proceed as follows:

1. Set up two basins—one with hot water, the other with cold water.

2. Sit in the hot-water basin first. Then sit in the cold-water basin.

The warm water relaxes the muscles around the anal sphincter and relieves spasms. Afterward, the cold water tightens the tissue.

Note, however that repeated immersion in hot water can temporarily impair male fertility.

# APPENDIX C

# Herbs

The practice of herbal healing goes back to the dawn of man. Ancient Egyptian and Chinese texts thousands of years old have recorded the use of herbs for treating and curing various ailments of the body, mind and spirit. Many of the plants used today in herbal medicine were used and described by Dioscorides, a first century Greek physician and botanist. His reference work "De Materia Medica," was for 1,500 years the standard work on botany and therapeutic use of plants.

The use of herbal teas, extracts and powders to help rebuild sickly and weak bodies is still used by virtually every culture. Many Native American communities used herbs for medicine, dyes, poisons and food. The Aztecs used nettles regularly and early American pioneers used lovage, sage, chives, lily of the valley, peppermint, thyme, flax, pennyroyal and chamomile. The English used dandelion and the Chinese, ginseng.

Today many herbs are used in modern medicine. Though many of these herbal remedies do not have a scientific basis as to why they work, they are the basis of some well known pharmaceuticals. It was the *cinchona* tree that gave us *quinine* for the treatment of malaria, the *foxglove plant* that gave us digitalis. Other herbs that are currently used by medical doctors in one form or another include red periwinkle, mayapple, witch hazel, and ginseng.

Though there is more sophisticated research on the value of herbal medicines than ever before, most of the information about herbs used in natural healing is based on the folklore passed down from generation to generation. Over the last fifteen years the use of herbal medicines in healing has increased to an amazing level. Herbal experts cite these major reasons why herbs have gained new found popularity: (1) many people desire to return to nature; (2) they fear the side effects associated with many over-the-counter and prescription drugs; (3) they are unhappy with the high cost and impersonal style of orthodox medicine; and (4) they've discovered that Indian, African, Asian and South American cultures have used herbal medicines with great success.

## Why Are Herbal Medicines Sometimes the Center of Controversy?

Many of the negative associations that medical doctors harbor towards herbal medicine are based on the fact that many commercially available herbal products are of poor quality. Some products do not even contain any of the herbs that are listed on the label.

This is especially true with ginseng formulas. To remedy this, many herb companies have formed trade associations in an attempt to upgrade the quality of their products.

As valuable as herbs are to the natural healing process, it is foolish to make believe that all herbal substances are free from danger. Many herbs contain deadly poisons, toxic substances or powerful alkaloids. Many herbs that may be of great medicinal value may be poisonous if used improperly and thus should never be used except under the guidance of a well trained herbalist or a physician who has a strong working knowledge of herbal medicines. The Food and Drug Administration has compiled a list of toxic herbs and their effects. A partial listing of these herbs is as follows.

| Potentially Toxic Herbs | Botanical Reference |
|---|---|
| Bittersweet | *Solanum dulcamara L.* |
| Horse Chestnut | *Sanguinaris canadensis* |
| Wahoo | *Euonymus atropurpureus* Jacq. |
| Deadly nightshade | *Atropa belladona L.* |
| European mandrake | *Mandragora officinarum L.* |
| Heliotrope | *Heliotropium europaeum L.* |
| Hemlock | *Conium maculatum L.* |
| Henbane | *Hyoscyamus niger L.* |
| Lobelia (Indian tobacco) | *Lobelia inflata L.* |
| Jalap root | *Exagonium purga* |
| Jimson weed | *Datura stramonium L.* |
| Lily of the valley | *Convallaria majalis L.* |
| May apple (American Mandrake) | *Podophyllum peltatum L.* |
| Mistletoe | *Phoradendron flavescens* (Pursh) |
| Morning glory | *Ipomoea purpurea (L.),* Roth |
| Periwinkle | *Vinca major L.* and *Vinca minor L.* |
| Pokeweed | *Phytolacca americana L.* |
| Scotch broom, Irish broom | *Cytisus scoparius (L.)* Link |
| Spindle tree | *Euonymus europaeus L.* |
| Sweet Flag | *Acorus calamus L.* |
| Tonka bean | *Dipteryx odorata* (Aubl.) Willd. |
| Water hemlock (Cowbane) | *Cicuta maculata L.* |
| Snakeroot | *Eupatorium rugosum Houtt* |
| Wolfsbane (Arnica) | *Arnica montana L.* |
| Wormwood (Mugwort) | *Artemosia absinthium* Linne |
| Yohimbe | *Corynanthe yohimbe* Schum. |

Some of the herbs on this list are dangerous, while others may be of benefit if used under the guidance of a properly trained clinician.

# Herbs as Healers

Among the most popular herbal healers used are:

*Aloe vera.* The gel of this plant may be applied topically to burns and other skin problems, and it is often taken orally as well. Aloe is often used in the southwestern United States and in Latin America for its antibacterial, antifungal and antiviral properties. In the Philipines, aloe vera gel is mixed with milk for the treatment of dysentery, intestinal infections and kidney problems. There are tribes in Zaire that use aloe for the treatment of ringworm and boils. Many healers use aloe gel for the treatment of digestive problems, arthritis and bursitis.

*Anise (Pimpinella anisum).* Anise may be boiled in milk to relieve gas pains and colic in small children. Anise tea is very soothing to the digestive tract.

*Astragalus (Astragalus membranaceus).* This is one of the most popular tonic herbs in oriental medicine. It has been used primarily to strengthen the immune system. Any disease or disorder that involved a breakdown or weakness of the immune system would call for astragalus as part of the total healing program.

*Arnica (Arnica montana).* This herb can be used as an external tincture for sprains and bruises.

*Bayberry bark (Myrica cerifera).* An excellent gargle for sore throats, bayberry is also used to clear congestion in the nose and sinuses.

*Black cohash root (Cimicifuga racemosa).* Used to reduce menopausal symptoms. Reduces pain of childbirth. Contains estrogen like substance.

*Black walnut hulls.* Used for many skin disorders. Expels parasites.

*Blessed thistle (Juglans nigra).* Useful for relieving migraine headaches. Valuable in many gynecological disorders.

*Blue cohash (Caulophyllus thalictroides).* Regulates menstrual flow. Used for heart palpitations and hypertension.

*Burdock root (Arctium lappa).* A blood cleanser and diuretic. It is also healing to the kidneys.

*Butcher's Broom (Ruscus aculeatus).* This herb is more popular in Europe than in the United States, but it is beginning to develop a strong following among natural healers due to it's anti-clotting and anti-inflammatory properties. It is most commonly used to treat various circulatory problems.

*Capsicum (Capsicum minimum).* This is common cayenne pepper. It is a catalyst for most other herbs. It is valuable for circulation, the heart and nerves.

*Catnip (Nepeta cataris).* Useful for children with colic, soothing to the nerves. Reduces pain from spasms.

*Chamomile (Anthemis nobilis).* Sedating to the entire nervous system. Reduces teething pain in children. Chamomile is used in many formulas for reducing stress.

*Chaparral (larrea tridentata; L. divaricata).* Used in many traditional herbal cancer treatment formulas. Used for arthritis, infections, acne and other sin conditions.

*Chickweed (Stellaria madia, Cyrill).* Used for swollen testes, hemorrhoids, bronchial problems.

*Comfrey (Symphytum officinale).* Available as a root or leaves. The root is most popular. Good for diarrhea, blood in urine, coughs and colds. Used to heal ulcers.

*Damiana (Turnera diffusa, Willd.).* Sexual rejuvenator and nerve stimulant.

*Dandelion root (Taraxacum officinale, Wiggers).* When used raw, it is a powerful diuretic; good for kidney and bladder problems.

*Echinacea (Echinacea angustifolia).* Used for all fevers and infections. Excellent blood cleanser.

*Eyebright (Euphrasia officinalis).* Used internally as a tea for problems of the eye, including conjunctivitis.

*Evening Primrose (Primula vulgaris, Huds.).* The oil of this plant is very high in certain hormone-like substances known as prostaglandins. Prostaglandins have been found to bring relief to a number of medical disorders.

*Fennel (Foeniculum vulgare).* Reduces flatulence and bloating from gas. Reduces colic in children. Good for digestion.

*Fo-Ti.* Helps memory and reduces depression. (A Chinese herb).

*Garlic (Allium sativum).* Garlic is an aid in healing all systemic infections, respiratory problems, and fever.

*Ginger (Zingiber officinale).* Reduces painful spasms of bowels and stomach. Used as a tea and in compresses. Ginger is one of the most popular herbs in Vietnamese medicine along with peppermint and eucalyptus.

*Ginseng (Pana quinquefolium).* Helps with nervous exhaustion, sexual function, poor circulation, loss of memory.

*Goldenseal root (Hydrastis canadensis).* One of the most popular herbs. Used to treat ulcers and most internal infections.

*Gotu kola.* Used in many nerve stimulant formulas.

*Hawthorn berries (Crataegus oxycantha).* Used for all heart problems.

*Horsetail (Equisetum arvense, Linn.).* Rich in silica. Helps skin healing and is a diuretic.

*Jojoba.* This desert shrub produces a wax-like substance (called jojoba oil) that is very similar to sperm whale oil. It is a highly versatile lubricant that is most useful in healing various skin and scalp disorders.

*Juniper berries (Juniperus communis).* Used in pancreatic, adrenal, bladder and kidney disorders. Especially useful in leucorrhea and edema.

*Licorice root (Glycyrrhiza glabra).* Soothing to the throat, licorice root contains a natural cortisone-like substance. Used for hypoglycemia, ulcers, stress and adrenal related problems.

*Lobelia (Lobelia inflata, Linn.).* The most powerful of all herbal relaxants. Reduces palpitation of the heart, fever. Note, however, this this herb should be used under the direction of a skilled herbalist.

*Marsh mallow root (Althaea officinalis, Linn.).* Bathe inflamed eyes in this tea. Good for problems of the lungs, kidneys, throat and digestion, especially diarrhea.

*Myrrh (Commiphora molmol).* Usually taken as tincture. Still used by many dentists. Used for ulcers, hemorrhoids, bronchial and lung disorders.

*Pau D'Arco (Taheebo).* Taheebo is the Indian name for the inner bark of the Tabebuia tree, found only the Andes mountains. This bark has been traditionally used by the Callaway tribe (descendants of the Incas). Taheebo contains a compound called *quechua*, a powerful antibiotic with virus-killing properties. The herb can be taken as a tea or in salve form. It has been used to reduce pain, to serve as a blood-builder, and to strengthen the immune response. Many healers claim that taheebo is effective in the treatment of candida, herpes and certain types of cancer. Limited research on the herb has been conducted in the United States, though it has become a popular healing herb in the last five years.

*Parsley (Carum petroselinum).* A powerful diuretic, rich in chlorophyll. Traditionally used for all gallbladder problems and for expelling stones.

*Peppermint (Mentha piperita).* Used for digestion and reducing fever. Use the cool tea to wash burns. It is high in tannic acid.

*Plantain (plantago major, Linn.).* Primarily used for menstrual disorders, plantain is also good for problems of the lungs, kidneys, throat and digestion especially, diarrhea.

*Psyllium (Plantago psyllium, Linn.).* Colon cleanser. Used in most detoxification programs.

*Red clover (Trifolium pratense, Linn.).* Relaxing for the nervous system. One of the best blood cleansers.

*Raspberry (Rubus idaeus, Linn.).* Relieves morning sickness in pregnancy. Strengthens the uterine wall prior to childbirth.

*Rosemary (Rosemarinus officinalis).* This pungent herb has been found in recent research to have the ability to act as an anti-oxidant and preservative in food. Because of it's strong odor and taste, it cannot easily be used in all foods.

*Saffron (Crocus sativus).* Aids digestion, arthritis and muscle fatigue.

*Sage.* Gargle with this tea to relieve a sore throat and ulcers in the mouth. Reduces involuntary sexual emissions in men (spermatorrhea). Expells worms. Also used for kidney and liver problems.

*Sarsparilla (Similax officinalis).* Blood cleanser.

*Sassafrass (Sassafras variifolium).* Used to ease colic and to heal skin eruptions. It was used by Native American tribes of the northeastern United States as a spring medicine to purify the blood.

*Scullcap (Scutellaria laterifolia, Linn.).* One of the best herbs for nervous disorders. It is used to reduce hypertension, heart problems and any problems of the central nervous system, including epilepsy.

*Siberian Ginseng (Eleutherococcus Senticosus).* This is not actually ginseng, but rather it is a member of the Araliaceae family of plants. Unlike other herbs this herb is not known for any particular curative effect but instead for restorative qualities. It is very valuable for people who are coming back from a health problem and are beginning to regain their strength.

*Slippery elm bark (Ulmus fulva).* This pleasant tasting herb was used by the native population and the early settlers in the form of poultices and liquids for the treatment of fevers and colds with cough. When treating an individual in a weak and debilitated condition, slippery elm supplies both a nutritive and gentle action on the body. Because of its mucilagenous quality, it is an ideal herb for tissue repair and is also known for its anti-inflammatory qualities.

*Thyme (Thymus vulgaris, Linn.).* Thyme can be used as an antiseptic and antispasmodic. Its aromatic essence is used to treat fevers and infections.

*Uva Ursi or Bearberry (Arctostaphylos uva-ursi).* Used in mature onset diabetes, kidney and bladder problems.

*Valerian root.* One of the best herbs for nervous disorders. Is used to reduce hypertension, heart problems and any problems of the central nervous system including epilepsy. Especially useful for sleep disorders.

*White oak bark.* Used for varicose veins and hemorrhoids. Normalizes the liver, kidney and spleen.

*White willow bark (Salix alba).* An Indian folk medicine which contains salicin, a prime ingredient in aspirin and a powerful anti-inflammatory agent, especially for arthritis.

*Yarrow.* Used for indigestion and run down conditions. If used at the beginning of a cold, it is very soothing to the mucous membranes and may break up the illness within 24 hours.

*Yellow dock.* Blood purifier and toner for the entire system. Very high in minerals.

*Yohimbe.* This herb is actually the bark of a tree that grows in Africa and Mexico. It has been used historically in tribal medicine as an aphrodisiac and sexual rejuvenator as well as a general remedy for impotency and other sexual dysfunctions. This herb should be used with caution and under the guidance of a trained herbalist or physician. Yohimbe is so strong a sexual stimulant that the hydrochloride derivative is a prescription drug.

*Yucca.* A desert plant that has shown some positive results in treating rheumatoid arthritis.

## The Ways Of Using Herbs

*Edible rice paper.* Carried by many health and nutrition stores.

*Alcohol bases, tinctures and extracts.* Many herbs are available in prepared extract form. Usually 20 to 30 drops of the extract are added to hot water. Various herbs can thus be easily mixed. These are preferred by many herbalists because they release the widest range of essential herbal healing elements in unaltered form. Alcohol-based formulas also permit faster sublingual absorption.

*Tea.* Take one ounce of herb tea. Add this to between six and eight ounces of boiled distilled water (turn the heat off before putting in the herb). Steep the herbs for 20 to 30 minutes and strain them out. Honey may be added to make some of the stronger teas more pleasant tasting. If preparing the tea from roots or bark, you can boil them for 20 to 30 minutes. Never boil the flowers or leaves.

*Food.* Such as slippery elm gruel.

*Poultices.* These are used (usually with a powdered herb) to cool, stimulate, or soothe irritated skin, ulcerations, boils, infected wounds and herpes eruptions, as well as for drawing out impurities through the skin. They are used as external applications, soft and pulpy; they should be applied warm or tepid, and should not be allowed to dry before being changed or renewed. Take the powdered herb and add some water to it and mix this into a paste. Place this moist powder into a porous cotton cloth or natural fiber cloth (this will keep it from drying onto the skin and hair. Place this on the area to be treated.

Some traditional poultices that have been used include:

• General poultice—Bread boiled in milk. Apples, pared, cored, and well boiled; mashed up into a pulp.

- Acute Pain—Green lettuce leaves, well boiled.
- Boils—Brown sugar and soap.
- Inflammations—Flax seed or chamomile flowers boiled with the tops of wormwood.

An alternate system for preparing a poultice is to take a few tablespoons of powder and place them in a flannel cloth dipped in boiling water for a minute or two. When the cloth has cooled, apply it to the affected area. Then when the cloth and herbs become too dry reimmerse them in the hot water. Be sure that the herbs you use are not harmful and are used appropriately. Some herbs when used in excess may be harmful.

# APPENDIX D

# Aroma Therapy

## Uses and Benefits of Essences

Plant essences have a threefold healing effect. First, the essence may have a soothing or an exciting effect. Your senses react to the aroma of the essence as you would to the aroma of a perfume or a flower. Second, the essence acts as a nerve stimulant by having a relaxing effect. Third, the chemical composition of each individual essence has its own unique effect.

Essences can be classified according to function:

• *Stimulating oils* include cardamon, cedar, cinnamon, fennel, lemon, and ylang-ylang. Such oils might be especially useful in, for example, cases of paralysis and loss of voice.

• *Sedating oils* include cajuput, chamomile, melissa, and peppermint. These might be used to help relieve insomnia and nervousness.

• *Antiseptic oils* include lemon, thyme, orange, bergamot, juniper, clove, citronella, lavender, niaouli, peppermint, rosemary, sandalwood, and eucalyptus. These oils are especially powerful when they are vaporized.

• *Antispasmodic oils* include lavender, marjoram, lemongrass, cypress, and anise.

## Specific Techniques

Aroma therapy can be employed in several different ways.

*By Room Dispersal.* You can effectively disperse an essence throughout a room by using a fine aerosol spray. If you have a reaction to other components in the spray, try this alternative method of room dispersal: Buy a small heat lamp with a crucible above the lamp. When you add several drops of an essence to the crucible, the heat will then disperse the essence throughout the room. Heat lamps are available at many of the places that sell essences.

*Topically.* Many essences are concentrated. Therefore, rather than apply them full strength, soak a compress in a diluted essence and apply the compress twice a day.

*By Friction Chest Rub.* Mix the essences in a base of lanolin and cocoa butter. Then rub the compound on your chest morning and night.

*Orally.* When you prepare an oral mixture, place about eight drops of each oil in a glass of lukewarm water. Be sure to combine no more than four or five oils and to use no more than 25 to 40 drops of all ingredients combined.

Take the mixture ten minutes before meals three times a day. For children, limit the dosage to three to ten drops three times a day.

Note that oils evaporate quickly when added to warm water. Also, some essences are too powerful to be taken orally.

Be sure to store essences in well-sealed, colored-glass containers, away from air and light. A good source for aromatic oils and dispersal equipment is:

Aroma Vera
P.O. Box 3609
Culver City, CA 90231
(213) 675-8219

# APPENDIX E

# Homeopathy

Homeopathy is among the most respected and effective natural healing approaches available. Though its principles are thousands of years old and were used in ancient India and Greece, its present form was discovered and applied in the early 1800s by a German physician, Samuel Christian Friedrich Hahnemann. Hahnemann derived the name homeopathy from the greek, *homoios* (similar) and *pathos* (suffering or sickness). The fundamental law that homeopathy is based on its known as the law of similars, or as it was described in latin "similia similibus curentur" (like is cured by like). This concept of healing states that a disease may be cured by a particular remedy if that remedy produced in a healthy person produces symptoms similar to those of the disease.

When you to to a homeopathic practitioner, you will be asked to describe all of your symptoms and you will be asked many questions about your own and your family's medical history. Once the homeopath has the essential information, he or she will search for a remedy that has been shown under scientifically controlled conditions to produce the same symptoms that your illness is characterized by, in a healthy person. By means of the law of similars, the homeopath is essentially selecting one remedy to produce a cure by matching your symptoms to the symptoms remedy induces.

Generally speaking the best way to use Homeopathy for any chronic condition is by working with a practitioner who is skilled in choosing the appropriate remedies. For acute conditions self treatment is appropriate and there is no chance of using the wrong remedy and creating an unwanted side effect.

## Dr. Schuessler's Cellular (Tissue Salt) Therapy

The use of homeopathically prepared tissue salts was pioneered by Wilhelm Heinrich Schuessler, a German medical doctor, physicist and physiological chemist. He developed this concept of healing in the early nineteenth century based on theories of his predecessor, Rudolph Virchow, a century before. Virchow discovered that the human body is made up of many tiny, living cells that are made up of water, organic substances, and inorganic substances. The inorganic substances, though present in very small quantities, were found to be essential to life. By Schessler's time it was known that if the blood lacked one of the inorganic elements, the rebuilding and healing processes in the body could not take place. According to Schuessler, deficiencies in these vital substances eventually lead to a disease state. In Schuessler's time only twelve inorganic elements had been isolated in the cellular matter. In modern times many more of these elements are known, however most healers still use the Cellular Therapy with the original twelve tissue salts with which Schuessler worked. They are listed below.

Calcium Fluoride (Calc. Fluor.)

Calcium Phosphate (Calc. Phos.)

Calcium Sulphate (Calc. Sulph.)

Phosphate of Iron (Ferr. Phos.)

Potassium Chloride (Kali. Mur.)

Potassium Phosphate (Kali. Phos.)

Potassium Sulphate (Kali. Sulph.)

Magnesium Phosphate (Mag. Phos.)

Sodium Chloride (Nat. Mur.)

Sodium Phosphate (Nat. Phos.)

Sodium Sulphate (Nat. Sulph.)

Silicic Oxide (Silica)

## The Bach Flower Remedies

Over 50 years ago, a young British scientist and physician named Edward Bach discovered that many of his patient's physical illnesses were directly related to certain emotional and psychological disturbances. Bach a pathologist, immunologist, and bacteriologist, noted that resentment, anxiety, worrisome thoughts, even lack of self-confidence so depleted a patient's vitality that the body lost its natural resistance and became susceptible to a host of organic illnesses. Today research in the field of psychoneuroimmunology supports these findings.

Following extensive research, Bach found that certain species of wildflowers, when picked at certain times in the blooming cycle and prepared homeopathically optimized the healing qualities of that plant. Bach eliminated those plants he found to be toxic or those which produced side-effects, and ultimately succeeded in discovering 38 flowering plants, trees and special waters which were found to have a profound affect in stabilizing a wide range of mental and emotional stresses. Unlike chemical drugs which can be suppressive and create dependency, the Bach Remedies, as they are known today, are considered completely safe, nonhabit-forming, and work by gently reestablishing emotional and psychological equilibrium.

Considered a major breakthrough, these preparations have been used for over 50 years by a broad spectrum of health care professionals worldwide, including medical doctors, dentists, chiropractors, and psychologists, as well as the general public. The remedies have also been used extensively by veterinarians and have been shown remarkably effective in alleviating fear and other emotional disturbances, as well as behavioral problems in animals.

*Rescue Remedy; the Emergency Remedy.* Rescue Remedy, the combination formula containing five of the Bach remedies, was developed and named by Dr. Bach for its calming and stabilizing effect in a broad range of emergency and traumatic situations. This includes, but is not limited to, the alleviation of acute stress arising from

# A Self Help Guide To
# The Bach Flower Remedies

The following indications have been reported in the standard Bach literature.

☐ **AGRIMONY**  For those not wishing to burden others with their troubles and who cover up their suffering behind a cheerful facade. They are distressed by argument or quarrel, and may seek escape from pain and worry through the use of drugs and alcohol.

☐ **ASPEN**  For those who experience vague fears and anxieties of unknown origin, they are often apprehensive.

☐ **BEECH**  For those who while desiring perfection easily find fault with people and things. Critical and at times intolerant, they may overreact to small annoyances or idiosyncrasies of others.

☐ **CENTAURY**  For those who are overanxious to please often weak willed and easily exploited or dominated by others. As a result they may neglect their own particular interests.

☐ **CERATO**  For those who lack confidence in their own judgment and decisions. They constantly seek the advice of others and may often be misguided.

☐ **CHERRY PLUM**  For fear of losing mental and physical control, of doing something desperate. May have impulses to do things thought or known to be wrong.

☐ **CHESTNUT BUD**  For those who fail to learn from experience, repeating the same patterns or mistakes again and again.

☐ **CHICORY**  For those who are overfull of care for others and need to direct and control those close to them. Always finding something to correct or put right.

☐ **CLEMATIS**  For those who tend to live in the future, lack concentration, are daydreamers, drowsy or spacey and have a halfhearted interest in their present circumstances.

☐ **CRAB APPLE**  For those who may feel something is not quite clean about themselves or have a fear of being contaminated. For feelings of shame or poor self image. For example, thinking oneself not attractive for one reason or another. When necessary, may be taken to assist in detoxification, for example, during a cold or while fasting.

☐ **ELM**  For those who at times may experience momentary feelings of inadequacy, being overwhelmed by their responsibilities.

☐ **GENTIAN**  For those who become easily discouraged by small delays or hindrances. This may cause self-doubt.

☐ **GORSE**  For feelings of hopelessness and futility. When there is little hope of relief.

☐ **HEATHER**  For those who seek the companionship of anyone who will listen to their troubles. They are generally not good listeners and have difficulty being alone for any length of time.

☐ **HOLLY**  To be used when troubled by negative feelings such as envy, jealousy, suspicion, revenge. Vexations of the heart, states indicating a need for more love.

☐ **HONEYSUCKLE**  For those dwelling in the past, nostalgia, homesickness, always talking about the good old days, when things were better.

☐ **HORNBEAM**  For the Monday morning feeling of not being able to face the day. For those feeling that some part of the body or mind needs strengthening. Constant fatigue and tiredness.

☐ **IMPATIENS**  For those quick in thought and action, who require all things to be done without delay. They are impatient with people who are slow and often prefer to work alone.

☐ **LARCH**  For those who despite being capable, lack self confidence or feel inferior. Anticipating failure they often refuse to make a real effort to succeed.

☐ **MIMULUS**  For fear of known things, such as heights, water, the dark, other people, of being alone, etc.

☐ **MUSTARD**  For deep gloom which comes on for apparently no known reason, sudden melancholia or heavy sadness. Will lift just as suddenly.

☐ **OAK**  For those who struggle on despite despondency from hardships, even when ill and overworked, they never give up.

☐ **OLIVE**  For mental and physical exhaustion, sapped vitality with no reserve. This may come on after an illness or personal ordeal.

☐ **PINE**  For those who feel they should do or should have done better, who are self-reproachful or blame themselves for the mistakes of others. Hardworking people who suffer much from the faults they attach to themselves, they are never satisfied with their success.

☐ **RED CHESTNUT**  For those who find it difficult not to be overly concerned or anxious for others, always fearing something wrong may happen to those they care for.

☐ **ROCK ROSE**  For those who experience states of terror, panic and hysteria, also when troubled by nightmares.

· ☐ **ROCK WATER**  For those who are very strict with themselves in their daily living. They are hard masters to themselves struggling toward some ideal or to set an example for others. This would include strict adherence to a living style or to religious, personal or social disciplines.

☐ **SCLERANTHUS**  For those unable to decide between two things, first one seeming right then the other. Often presenting extreme variations in energy or mood swings.

☐ **STAR OF BETHLEHEM**  For grief, trauma, loss. For the mental and emotional effect during and after a trauma.

☐ **SWEET CHESTNUT**  For those who feel they have reached the limits of their endurance. For those moments of deep despair when the anguish seems to be unbearable.

☐ **VERVAIN**  For those who have strong opinions and who usually need to have the last word, always teaching or philosophizing. When taken to an extreme they can be argumentative and overbearing.

☐ **VINE**  For those who are strong willed. Leaders in their own right who are unquestionably in charge. However, when taken to an extreme they may become dictatorial.

☐ **WALNUT**  Assists in stabilizing emotional upsets during transition periods, such as puberty, adolescence and menopause. Also helps one to break past links and emotionally adjust to new beginnings such as moving, changing or taking a new job, beginning or ending a relationship.

☐ **WATER VIOLET**  For those who are gentle, independent, aloof and self-reliant, who do not interfere in the affairs of others, and when ill or in trouble prefer to bear their difficulties alone.

☐ **WHITE CHESTNUT**  For constant and persistent unwanted thoughts, such as, mental arguments, worries or repetitious thoughts that prevent peace-of-mind, and disrupt concentration.

☐ **WILD OAT**  For the dissatisfaction with not having succeeded in one's career or life goal. When there is unfulfilled ambition, career uncertainty or boredom with one's present position or station in life.

☐ **WILD ROSE**  For those, who for no apparent reason, have resigned themselves to their circumstances. Having become indifferent, little effort is made to improve things or find joy.

☐ **WILLOW**  For those who have suffered some circumstance or misfortune, which they feel was unfair or unjust. As a result they become resentful and bitter toward life or toward those who they feel were at fault.

NOTE: Conditions requiring proper medical attention should be referred to a physician.

© Copyright 1984 Bach Centre USA.

accidents, bereavement, hysteria, and times of fright. Even minor stresses, such as arguments, the anxiety over taking exams, making speeches, job interviews, and other similar situations are reportedly helped with Rescue Remedy.

Dr. Jerry Mittleman, a New York City dentist keeps a dropper bottle of Rescue Remedy by each chair in his office. He gives the patient a few drops of the remedy before beginning his treatment. He's found that Rescue Remedy helps raise the patient's resistive capacity to stress, while at the same time having a great calming influence.

In addition to a liquid concentrate, Rescue Remedy also comes in a cream which is said to be extremely useful in reducing pain and swelling when applied to bruises, bumps, sprains, minor burns, cuts, insect bites, and hemorrhoids. Using the liquid Rescue Remedy orally in conjunction with Rescue Remedy cream is also said to ease emotional upset associated with the aforementioned conditions. Additionally, this cream is also said to be effective in reducing pain, when applied to tension headaches, and acute muscle tension and stiffness.

Despite its diverse application, Rescue Remedy is not meant to take the place of emergency medical treatment, but it is reported to stabilize emotions such as fear and panic which often accompany these traumatic situations.

## Resources for Homeopathy and Cellular Therapy (Tissue Salts)

Homeopathic Educational Services
5916 Chabot Crest
Oakland, CA 94618

National Center For Homeopathy
1500 Massachusetts NW #41
Washington, D.C. 20005

International Foundation for
 Homeopathy
1141 N.W. Market
Seattle, WA 98107

United States Homeopathic
 Association
6560 Blacklick Road
Springfield, VA 22150

## Recommended Reading

The Science Of Homeopathy, By George Vithoulkas. Published by Grove Press, Inc. New York, 1980.

Homeopathic Medicine at Home, By Maesimund B. Panos, M.D. and Janee Heimlich. Published by J. P. Tarcher, Inc. Los Angeles, 1980

Homeopathic Remedies; For Physicians, Laymen and Therapists, By David Anderson, M.D., Dale Buegel M.D., and Dennis Chernin, M.D. Published by Himalayan Institute, Honesdale 1978

Biochemic Theory and Practice by J. B. Chapman, M.D. and Edward L. Perry M.D. Now available as The Biochemic Handbook, Published by Formur Inc. St. Louis

How To Use The Twelve Tissue Salts, By Esther Chapman, Jove/HBJ, 1977

Biochemistry Up To Date, by Eric F. Powell, Published by Health Science Press 1963, England.

## Homeopathic Pharmacies

Boericke and Tafel, Inc.
1011 Arch Street
Philadelphia, PA 19107
(215) 922-2967

Ehrhart and Karl, Inc.
17 Wabash Avenue
Chicago, IL 60602
(312) 332-1046

Luyties Pharmacal Company
4200 Laclede Avenue
St. Louis, MO 63108
1-800-325-8080

Washington Homeopathic Pharmacy
4914 Delray Avenue
Bethesda, MD 20014
(301) 656-1695

Humphreys Pharmacal, Inc.
63 Meadow Road
Rutherford, NJ 07070
(201) 933-7744

John A. Borneman and Sons
1208 Amosland Road
Norwood, PA 19074
(215) 532-2035

Standard Homeopathic Pharmacy
436 West 8th Street
Los Angeles, CA 90014
(213) 321-4284

# APPENDIX F

# Bodyworks

## The Basic Techniques of Bodywork

This section will concentrate on three basic techniques of bodywork, out of many hundreds of techniques that exist. The three are general rhythmic pressure, circular rhythmic pressure, and kneading.

Before you begin, it is important to be aware that if certain medical conditions exist, some bodywork techniques are not recommended. If you have any of the following listed physical conditions, be aware that caution should be exercised, including checking with your physician before having a massage that uses deep pressure or manipulation.

heart condition

hypertension

unhealed bone fractures

osteoporosis

fever

bone, muscle or skin disease including active infections under the skin

recently torn tendons, ligaments or muscles

diabetes

cancerous tumor

tubercular joints

thrombosis (an obstruction in a blood vessel, caused by clotting of the blood

acute inflammation (bodywork may be used on uninflamed parts

skin disease in any form except thickened skin left by chronic eczema

aneurisms (dilation of an artery)

osteoarthritis when there is danger of fracturing

osteoarthritis when there is active inflammation (signs are heat, redness and soreness)

frostbite

acute inflammation of the kidneys

## General Rhythmic Pressure

The two types of rhythmic pressure are general and circular. Rhythmic pressure is used to relieve deep-rooted muscle tension, structural problems, restrictions in the range of motion, in addition to pinpointing energy blockages. Rhythmic pressure is especially effective for muscle spasms and cramps, and in addition is one of the primary techniques in use to heal damaged tissue and prevent excessive scar tissue following surgery or sprains.

*Step 1.* Using your thumb, find the center of the "knot" in the muscle, or the tightness. You will probably find it especially sensitive.

*Step 2.* Press your thumb into the area around the discomfort, using the weight of your body. Hold for one to three seconds, then release; repeat. Continue in this manner as you move around the affected area. Move clockwise. Be sure to lift your thumb between each pressure, rather than sliding it along the skin. (In some situations the heel of the hand is better, and needs to be determined one case at a time.)

*Caution:* This technique is not to be used when the body temperature is above or below normal.

When applying pressure, even deep pressure, be sure to increase the pressure gradually—never suddenly. Do not push forcefully with your finger. Use the weight of your body to increase the pressure gradually.

## Circular Rhythmic Pressure

Slowly press your thumb down on the area where there is pain, spasm or limited motion. Rotate your thumb on this area in a clockwise motion. Be careful not to slide your thumb across the skin or lift it off the area. Simply revolve it slowly in one spot while manipulating the underlying tissue. As you move your thumb in a circular direction, begin to slowly increase the pressure. (This may be a little uncomfortable but never work deeply enough to cause extreme pain.)

As you continue this motion, you will find the pain and spasm slowly disappearing. You may also feel a sensation of heat or pulsation in your thumb. Sometimes this sensation is the pulse beat in your thumb but not always. Acupressure teachers often speak of this sensation as an opening up of an energy blockage.

Remember, never increase the pressure suddenly. It is the gradual pressure that creates the healing response. This technique should not be applied in a case of extreme swelling and inflammation.

## Kneading

This technique, which is similar to kneading bread dough, is used to stimulate the functions of the skin. It is especially effective with very dry skin, as it stimulates the vital functions of the parts of the body at the point of application, including nerves, blood vessels and glands, as well as muscles and connective tissue.

The body experiences kneading as alternation between compression and relaxation. By helping to empty the blood and lymph vessels, it brings fresh fluid into these areas, thereby improving circulation while eliminating poisons and waste matter from the tissues.

*Step 1.* Apply a small film of oil on the area to be worked on, then grasp the muscle with a squeezing action of your hand. With the proper amount of oil, the muscle will immediately start to slip out of your hand.

*Step 2.* As this happens, quickly grasp the muscle. It will continue to slide from hand to hand as you press it, and a rolling effect is created. On most areas, continue this kneading procedure for approximately thirty seconds to one minute. For the back, continue for about five minutes.

# Acupressure Chart A

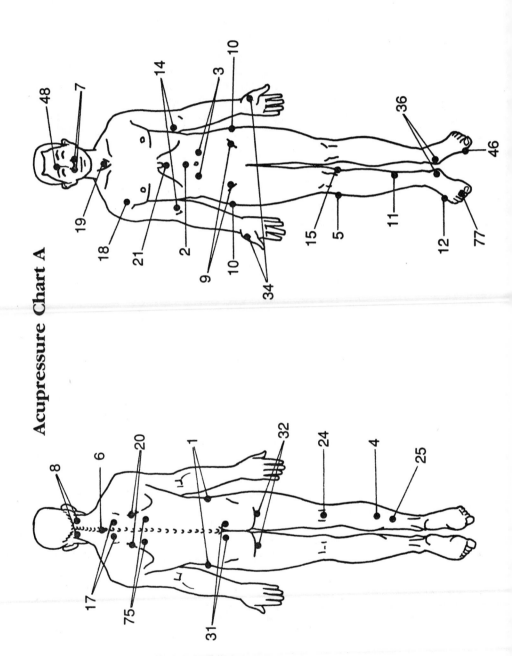

# Acupressure Chart B

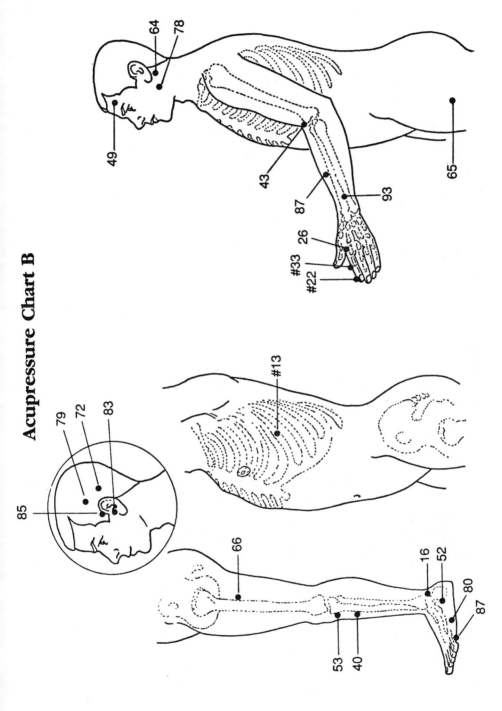

# Acupressure Chart C

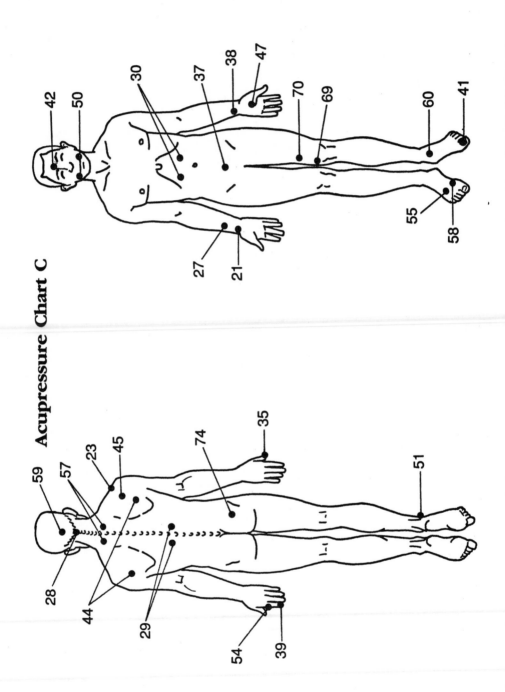

# Acupressure Chart D

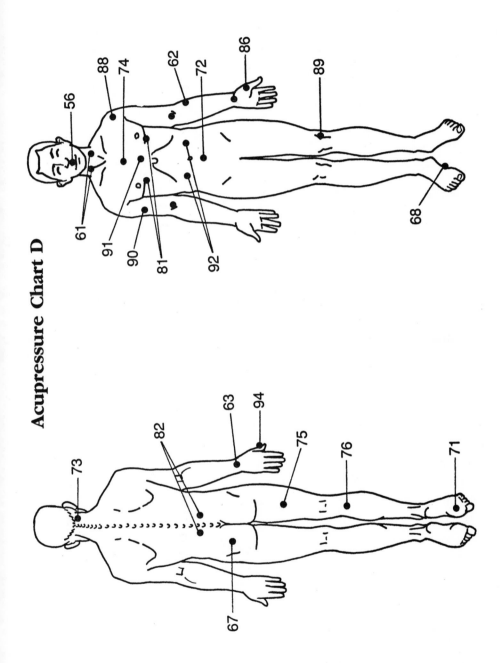

|                | **A**                    | **B**              | **C**                        | **D**        |
|----------------|--------------------------|--------------------|------------------------------|--------------|
| Allergies      | 6, 7, 8, 36              |                    |                              |              |
| Ankle pain     | 10, 11, 12               |                    |                              |              |
| Arm pain       | 14                       | 33                 |                              | 88, 89, 90   |
| Arthritis      | 2, 4, 5                  | 13, 26, 16         |                              | 89, 90       |
| Asthma         | 17, 19, 18, 20           |                    |                              | 91           |
| Bronchitis     | 14, 6, 18                |                    | 21                           | 92, 74       |
| Bursitis       | 21, 14                   |                    | 39, 23                       | 88           |
| Calf pain      | 4, 24                    |                    |                              |              |
| Cold           | 7, 25, 8, 17, 18         | 26                 | 73, 27, 28                   |              |
| Colitis        | 3, 31                    | 40                 | 29, 27, 30                   |              |
| Constipation   | 32, 3, 31, 11, 9         | 26, 33, 93         |                              | 92           |
| Cough          | 34, 75, 36, 17, 11       |                    | 57, 27                       | 94           |
| Cystitis       | 15, 31                   |                    | 29, 37, 70                   |              |
| Dental pain    |                          |                    | 38, 39                       |              |
| Diarrhea       | 3, 2, 31                 | 26, 40             | 27, 54                       | 68           |
| Dizziness      |                          |                    | 58, 42                       |              |
| Elbow pain     | 14                       | 26, 43             | 23                           | 62           |
| Fatigue        | 14                       |                    | 45, 23, 41                   |              |
| Sore eyes      | 48                       | 26                 | 54                           | 73           |
| Facial pain    |                          | 26, 78             | 50, 51                       |              |
| Foot pain      | 12, 36, 11               | 87, 80, 52, 16     | 51                           | 76           |
| Foot pain      | 11                       | 52                 | 51                           |              |
| Gallbladder    |                          | 52                 | 30, 29                       |              |
| Gastritis      | 3, 17, 2, 53             |                    | 44                           |              |
| Gingivitis     |                          | 26                 | 50, 35                       |              |
| Gout           |                          |                    | 54, 55                       |              |
| Hand pain      |                          |                    | 23, 44                       |              |
| Hayfever       |                          | 26                 | 57, 28                       | 56           |
| Headache       | 8                        |                    | 27, 21, 58, 59, 57, 26       |              |
| Hiccups        | 2, 5, 21                 |                    | 29                           |              |
| High blood pressure | 2                   |                    | 60                           | 61           |
| Indigestion    | 12, 9, 3                 |                    | 30                           | 62           |
| Influenza      | 11, 6                    |                    | 57                           | 63           |

| | A | B | C | D |
|---|---|---|---|---|
| Insomnia | 11 | 64, 65 | | 61 |
| Knee pain | 15, 5 | | | |
| Leg pain | 4, 32, 5, 15 | 53, 40, 65 | | |
| Low blood pressure — | | 66 | 28 | |
| Lower back pain | 24 | 16 | 51 | 67 |
| Menstrual irregularity | 11 | | 37 | 68, 70 |
| Menstrual pain | | 66 | 70 | 21, 71 |
| Stress (mental) | 20 | | 42, 28, 21, 57 | |
| Migraine headache | | 26, 72, 64 | 37, 21, 38, 28, 3 | 73 |
| Motion sickness | 2, 21 | 75 | 42 | 74 |
| Nasal congestion | 17, 8, 7, 12 | | 42 | |
| Nausea | 2, 5, 11, 72, 9 | | 29, 27 | 68 |
| Neck pain | 17, 12 | 64, 72 | 44 | 73 |
| Sciatica | 32, 4 | 16 | 74, 51 | 75, 76 |
| Shoulder pain | | 43 | 23, 44, 45 | |
| Sinus problems | 77, 7 | 26, 78 | 42 | 56 |
| Sore throat | | 26 | 35 | |
| Stiff neck | | 78, 79, 80 | 28, 23 | 73 |
| Stomach pain | 75 | 40 | 30, 29, 37 | 81, 72 |
| Tennis elbow | | 26, 43 | 44 | 82 |
| Tinnitus | 8 | 83, 85, 26 | | 61 |
| Tonsillitis | 5 | 26, 87, 78 | | 86 |
| Toothache | 77 | 16, 33, 64, 83 | | |
| Whiplash | 19, 8 | 26 | 44, 57 | |
| Earache | | 26 | | |
| Fainting | | | 38 | 71 |
| Hemorrhage | 14, 36 | | | 63 |
| Testicle pain | | | | 68 |
| Wound pain | | 87 | 23, 69 | |
| Reducing hunger | | 83 | | |

# Index